Safety for Stalking Victims

Safety for Stalking Victims

How to save your *privacy*, your *sanity*, and your *life*

Lyn Bates

Writer's Showcase
San Jose New York Lincoln Shanghai

Safety for Stalking Victims
How to save your privacy, your sanity, and your life

Writer's Showcase
an imprint of iUniverse.com, Inc.

For information address:
iUniverse.com, Inc.
5220 S 16th, Ste. 200
Lincoln, NE 68512
www.iuniverse.com

ISBN: 0-595-18160-0

Printed in the United States of America

To Roger, for everything.

Contents

* ❖ *What is stalking?*
* ❖ *Who are stalking victims?*
* ❖ *Necessary and unnecessary fear*
* ❖ *Who stalks?*
* ❖ *Types of stalkers*
* ❖ *"Why me?"*
* ❖ *"It's not fair!"*
* ❖ *"So, how much danger am I in?"*
* ❖ *Relaxed awareness*

* ❖ *Take responsibility for your own safety*
* ❖ *"He's trying to drive me crazy, and I'm not going to give him the satisfaction!"*
* ❖ *"I'm not going to give in to my fear!"*
* ❖ *How to prevent stalking from starting*
* ❖ *As soon as you* think *you might have a problem*
* ❖ *As soon as you* know *you have a problem*
* ❖ *Take control*

Foreword

Stalking has become a national epidemic. Across the country, 1.4 million Americans are stalked each year. They're followed everywhere they go—to work, to the market, to their health club, to their place of worship, to their home—until they don't feel safe anywhere. They receive an unending stream of phone calls or letters that range from proclamations of undying love to threats that "if I can't have you, no one can." Property is vandalized. Physical assaults are sometimes perpetrated. Friends and loved ones are targeted or threatened as well. In short, fear becomes a constant companion. With a rising sense of panic, stalking targets look for help. There's not much to be found in the traditional arenas to which they turn.

Despite the staggering numbers, few resources detail the dangers of stalking or offer solutions to this burgeoning problem. Which means that stalking targets must shoulder the responsibility for their own well-being. That's not an easy task in the best of circumstances. But it can be downright debilitating when your ordinary life has literally been blown apart, often by someone you know and trusted at some point along the way.

Though novels, television shows and movies would have us believe that strangers lurk in the shadows waiting to stalk us, most stalkings are conducted by people we were once close to. The husband who abused his wife during their marriage is not about to relinquish his sense of power if and when she finally screws up enough courage to leave him. So he resorts to another form of domestic violence: he stalks her.

His actions may change but the intent remains the same: to control another person's life through fear. The more scared his target becomes, the easier and more satisfying his mission. Worse, since most stalkers try to control their victims by isolating them, stalking victims often feel that they're completely alone. The growing sense of helplessness and hopelessness that ensues also serves the stalker well.

If you think this doesn't—and won't ever—apply to you, think again. The National Institute of Justice estimates that one out of every 12 women, and one out of every 20 men, will be stalked in their lifetimes. When I was researching *Surviving A Stalker: Everything You Need To Know To Keep Yourself Safe* (Marlowe & Co., 2000), I discovered just how close to home stalking hit in my own life. Though they'd never said a word, a number of my friends had been targeted by former mates, co-workers, or even strangers they'd had the misfortune of attracting. Indeed, it seems that every third person I tell about my book has either been stalked or knows someone who has. Their stories share the same pattern of escalation, and the same range of reactions: feelings of flattery or incredulity quickly change to irritation, apprehension, and, eventually, the debilitating sense of losing control over their lives.

Regaining that control is critical. Sadly, however, the natural reactions of most stalking victims put—and keep—them at a disadvantage. For starters, most usually can't believe that they're being stalked. The most common question voiced in the online support group located on the Stalking Victims' Sanctuary website (www.stalkingvictims.com) is: Am I being stalked? The details provided leave no doubt as to the inappropriate attention being directed towards them. But by denying the problem and not taking appropriate steps to protect their privacy and safety, they've already given their stalker the upper hand. Allowing him to isolate them emotionally just makes things worse.

If you've been targeted by a stalker, it's up to you to reclaim your life. The police aren't going to be able to do that for you. Neither are your family or friends. They can all support your actions. They may even be able to provide you with help. But in the end, you're going to have to count on yourself. Which means that you'll want to arm yourself with as much information as possible. You'll want to stay connected with others going through similar situations, so you can lean on them and learn from their triumphs and their mistakes. And you'll want to take the necessary precautions to safeguard your privacy and safety.

Whether you're looking to protect yourself from someone who's stalking you now, or you're simply seeking to prevent someone from targeting you in the future, Lyn Bates' encyclopedic *Safety for Stalking Victims: How to Save your Privacy, your Sanity and your Life* is a must. You won't want to take all of the precautions she lists. You don't need to. But knowing about your options and following those security measures that feel right and apply to you can help you reclaim your life...and could even save it.

You can take your power back. More power to you!

Linden Gross

Linden Gross is the author of *Surviving a Stalker: Everything You Need to Know to Keep Yourself Safe* (Marlowe & Co., 2000). She is the creator of The Stalking Victims' Sanctuary, located at www.stalkingvicitms.com. And she is the founder and president of Stalking Survivors' Sanctuary & Solutions, a non-profit organization dedicated to educating people about stalking and how to cope with it, and to furthering understanding about the problem's dynamics and possible solutions.

Preface

When Elizabeth McCandless Murray left her extremely abusive husband after only a year of marriage, he told her "If you leave me, I'll kill you stone-dead." Betsy believed him. Sean had tried to control every aspect of her life. He would not let her visit her mother. He even threw away her address book to limit her outside contacts. Betsy tried to get the police and the criminal justice system to protect her. She got a restraining order. He violated it 13 times. She even took a self-defense course, but nobody told her that the course was designed to deflect rapists, not murders. She left her high tech job and tried to go into hiding. But when he finally found her, he kept his promise. He shot her dead.

I cringed when I read that story. Here was a woman who knew she was in danger, and wanted to protect herself. Probably a great many well-meaning people had told her "Be careful" with true concern, but without telling her how to be careful, because they didn't know themselves how to protect against a smart, angry, twisted person who was absolutely determined to end Betsy's life, and then his own.

Betsy probably didn't know that Sean's attempts to contact her after their divorce constituted stalking. She probably didn't know that many women who are murdered are stalked before they are killed, whether they have a prior relationship with their murders or not. Although Betsy was trying hard to protect herself, nobody gave her the information or training that could have saved her life.

When I helped to start We are AWARE, an organization dedicated to teaching women about effective self-protection, I thought the worst situations we would deal with would be women wanting to protect themselves against rape. Wrong. Rape is one of the most common crimes against women, but it isn't necessarily the worst. Stalking can go on for years, continually terrifying the victim. Regardless of whether a stalking target reacts with intense bravado or pulls into a self-imposed shell, the unrelenting stress of a stalker's attentions can produce serious physical and psychological consequences.

It is not a rare problem—one out of every 12 women, and one out of every 20 men, will be stalked sometime in their life, according to the National Institute of Justice. Most of those episodes end well. Some of them don't. It's important to learn to judge when nuisance turns to danger, and what to do right from the beginning to reduce the chance of that happening. And if you're already being stalked, it's critical to learn what you can do to reduce the danger.

As a competitive shooter and a certified firearms instructor, I always wondered why there so little mention of the utility of guns for self-protection. As the vice president of AWARE, I know that women need a range of options to deal with danger, not just firearms. And the more training that they receive, the more intelligent the choices they can make to defend themselves. The profits from this book will go directly to AWARE, to enable us to reach even more people in danger.

You'll find in this book a wide range of options discussed ranging from firearms, to knives, to pepper spray, to the modern equivalent of brass knuckles, the Persuader keychain. You'll learn to examine self-defense classes to make sure that they teach you the right skills to get yourself out of trouble. And you'll learn what the best practices are, by police and prosecutors around the country, and how they are helping stalking victims.

Besides reading this book, I encourage you to find back issues of *Women&Guns* magazine, where over one hundred of my articles will tell you about full impact self-defense fighting, knife defense, defensive driving, and improvised weapons.

Using force when necessary means using judgment. The places where I went to develop my judgment were Lethal Force Institute, in

Concord New Hampshire, and other top firearms schools. The place where I went to test my judgment was the annual National Tactical Invitational, where I and other private citizens competed with local and federal law enforcement officers and some military folk in extremely realistic scenarios. SWAT team cops played the part of bad guys, and we were scored based on our shooting ability, as well as tactics, judgment, and our ability to verbally interact with the role players, using words whenever possible instead of bullets.

I am not an athlete, and I'm certainly not a police officer. What I am is an ordinary woman who has become more than ordinarily able to protect herself. And in this book I'll teach you much of what I've learned.

More and more people are contacting AWARE when they face the challenge of protecting themselves. Some of those people came because they were being stalked, or had been at one time. These people had made the decision to take what some people might call "extreme" measures to protect themselves. But as I write this, I'm glad to say that all of those "extreme" individuals are still alive today.

But newspaper stories tell a far more depressing tale of women who did not understand the danger they were in, or did not know how to deal with it. Some of those women died at the hands of their stalkers.

If you're being stalked, or just harassed and annoyed, you can't put your defense in the hands of someone else. The legal process can take years, and police procedures can vary widely across the country. Your safety has to rest primarily in your own hands. Too often you're told to "be careful" without being told HOW to "be careful." And that's why you're reading this book. Because here you're going to learn how to put the odds on your side rather than on your stalker's. Which is just where they ought to be!

Acknowledgements

Some people have provided information for this book, and would prefer to remain anonymous. They are stalking victims from whom I have learned a lot, whose plights clarified the need for a book like this, and whose privacy I will respect by not identifying them.

My fellow board members of the non-profit group AWARE, whose mission is to inform women about effective means of self-protection, deserve much credit for the information presented here and on AWARE's web site, www.aware.org.

In particular, Barbara Clorite and Jana Gabarro of AWARE provided useful feedback on early drafts of this document, and their input has strengthened it. Melissa Soalt, of PowerPact Inc. had many useful comments, particularly about the sections on fighting. Peggy Hanly, a domestic violence and stalking survivor who does not seek anonymity, provided many helpful comments and suggestions from her personal experience. Roger Lanny provided continual support and encouragement, as well as feedback. Mary Van Deusen is the best friend and editor anyone could hope to have.

And in the course of doing background work for this document, I learned a great deal from the works of Gavin de Becker, Linden Gross, Reid Meloy, Paul Mullen, Michele Pathe and Rosemary Purcell, Melita Schaum and Karen Parrish, Michael Scott, and the others whose books are in the reading list.

Responsibility for errors and omissions is entirely my own. If you find any as you use this book, or if you have suggestions of your own for the next edition, please let me know—you can send email to bates@aware.org, or contact me through AWARE, whose address and phone number are in Appendix A.

Introduction

As a stalking victim, you are suddenly and unexpectedly deprived of the sense of safety and security that you always had, and took for granted. The result is often profound fear, or at least a life-changing, uncomfortable awareness of vulnerability.

Knowledge is power, knowledge is safety, and you can learn everything you need to know to take care of yourself. This book is the first step.

❖ Who This Book Is For

This book is primarily intended for people, women or men, who are being victimized by stalkers. Since women stalking victims substantially outnumber men (the Department of Justice reports that 8% of women and 2% of men have been stalked), a few sections are relevant to women only, but most steps to safety are exactly the same for either men or women.

This book also contains information that will be valuable to those who want to avoid becoming victims of this devastating crime.

Finally, this book is intended for those who want to assist people who are being stalked in their quest for safety—friends, family, co-workers, police, prosecutors, workers in social service agencies, and others.

❖ *Safety, Not Justice*

Many issues about stalkers and stalking are beyond the scope of this book. We do not get into discussions here about the theories of what turns some people into stalkers, or how to prevent people from becoming stalkers. Nor do we have much to say about how to get justice through the justice system.

This book concentrates on one thing and one thing only: safety.

Safety is what you need, and you can get it! It is almost entirely in your control! "Justice," on the other hand, is mostly under the control of other people, which is why you cannot always get it.

❖ *Don't* feel *safe*. Be *safe!*

The goal of this book is not to make you *feel* safe. It is to make you *be* safe. Those are quite different things.

I have heard too many people recommend that a someone who is being stalked should take a self-defense course, because it will make them "feel safer." Unfortunately, a false sense of security is exactly what can happen if you take most "self-protection" courses that are oriented towards protection from rape.

Don't get me wrong. A good rape-prevention course is excellent protection against rape, but most stalkers aren't rapists. As a stalking victim, you need very specific information that is relevant to the crime that you are enduring, not some other crime.

Protecting yourself means more than just keeping your stalker away. It means having the skill, and the will, to take care of yourself in virtually any circumstances.

This book has hundreds of concrete suggestions. Nobody needs them all—you should choose the ones that best fit your situation. They will actually increase your safety. And after you *are* safer, you will start to *feel* safer again.

1 Stalking, Fear, and Danger

It started with an invitation to dinner. Or perhaps it began with a gift of flowers from an anonymous admirer. Or maybe it began with a peculiar letter from a "fan." Or maybe it started with the growled threat, "You can't leave me, bitch!"

However it started, you now feel uncomfortable every time the phone rings, every time you have to be out alone at night, every time you go to your car or reach for your mail. He is out there, somewhere, and his unceasing, unwanted attentions make your skin crawl and your hands clammy.

You never thought it would happen to you, but you are being stalked.

Stalking is an insidious crime that eats away at your sense of security, leaving you feeling more vulnerable than ever before in your life.

❖ What is stalking?

Fundamentally, stalking is a pattern of willful, malicious, unwelcome attention or behavior that makes you concerned or afraid. You might be afraid for your own safety or your family's safety. The stalker must commit more than one act of unwanted harassment, pursuit, intrusion, or communication. If someone seems obsessively persistent, "won't take NO for an answer," he (or she) is probably a stalker.

The actual behaviors that stalkers use are as varied as their personalities.

1

Some stalkers make unwanted phone calls which can be pleasant or unpleasant, frequent or occasional, demanding, pleading, questioning, or threatening.

Others write letters, which can also run the gamut in frequency and tone.

Some leave "gifts" ranging from the traditional (flowers, candy) to the bizarre (damaged photographs, a bedpan).

Stalkers may order pizza, taxis, or other services to be delivered to the homes of their targets. They have been known to cancel essential services in their victim's name, such as telephone or electricity.

Some stalkers use email, on-line chat groups, or other computer aids to carry out their harassment.

Others physically follow their prey, staying hidden or brazenly allowing themselves to be seen. Keeping the target of their obsession under surveillance, particularly at home, is a common technique.

Some break into homes, vandalize property, make threats, or kill pets.

A few attempt rape, kidnapping, or murder, and some succeed.

Melita Schaum, a stalking expert who co-authored a book on stalking with Karen Parrish, says, "…stalking is disordered, sick, and abnormal. It is essentially violent, abusive, antisocial behavior not acceptable or justifiable under any circumstances."

Stalking is much more common than most people think. The best estimates available at this time indicate that around 12% of women and 4% of men can expect to be stalked sometime in their lives.

Stalking is now illegal in every state, but laws vary widely from state to state about what exactly qualifies as stalking. Often, for a stalker's actions to be illegal, these 3 criteria must all be met:

1. The stalker must deliberately carry out a series of actions against you, the stalking victim, that would cause a reasonable person to fear bodily injury or death.

2. The stalker must know, or should have known, that you would be afraid as a result of his actions. That is, he must intend to cause you fear or harm.

3. You must truly be afraid of injury or death as a result of the stalker's actions.

That first requirement means that the stalker must *intentionally* direct his actions toward you. Someone who *accidentally* happened to cross your path several times a day would not be a stalker, even if he frightened you.

Also, it means that the stalker has to carry out a series of actions over time. No single incident can qualify as stalking.

Finally, that first requirement means that a "reasonable person" in your shoes would also be afraid. This "reasonable person" standard appears in many laws; it is there to prevent innocent people from being accused by a fraudulent victim or by a person with an unusually low tolerance for behavior that others do not find objectionable. This is where many cases fail to pass the legal requirement. It is often hard for "reasonable people" who aren't in your situation to understand why receiving flowers, letters, and phone calls from someone is making you afraid.

If the stalker tries to get at you through threatening other people in your family or household, that is also illegal in many states.

Stalking is hard to define, because everyone has a different opinion. Victims have one set of criteria for what they find terrifying, psychologists and psychiatrists have different criteria based on diagnostic categories and potential treatments, and police and courts have yet a different way of defining what is and isn't stalking, based on what must be proven in court.

Even if what you are experiencing doesn't meet your state's formal legal definition of stalking, you should still do all you can do to provide for your safety.

❖ *Who are stalking victims?*

If you are being stalked, you are probably a woman; 80% of stalking victims are female. If you are a man being stalked, it is likely that your stalker will be another man, possibly a neighbor, friend, or professional acquaintance.

Commonly, victims are between 18 and 29 years old when the stalking begins, but they can be any age from children to very senior citizens. They can be any sex, nationality, race or socioeconomic class.

Most, but not all, victims are well acquainted with their stalker. There was often an intimate relationship, a professional acquaintance, or a casual friendship.

If you are in the public eye, you may be stalked by someone who likes you a lot, or by someone who hates you. If you work for a political or social organization that generates a lot of opposition, someone who disagrees with your group's views might stalk you. Someone who wants to get revenge for being fired or for perceived mistreatment may stalk not just managers, but other people in the company.

If you are a member of the helping professions (medical, legal, educational, social work, etc.), you are particularly at risk for stalkers from the population you encounter as patients, students, and clients.

• **The V word**

A word on terminology here. In this book I will use the word "victim" to refer to people who are being stalked. Why not use a gentler term, like "stalking target"?

Unlike rape, which is usually over in minutes or hours, stalking is a crime that goes on for months or years. If you were raped, that happened in the past, and you survived the experience, so it is accurate to call you a rape survivor; you were only a rape victim during the time of the attack.

However, if you are being stalked, the crime is still going on, and you are still being victimized. You cannot truly be a "stalking survivor" until the stalking ends.

There is another reason to use the term "stalking victim." Stalking was not a crime anywhere in the United States until 1990, and in most states stalking statues are much more recent. So, prior to that time, people who were the targets of a stalker's fear-inducing, disgusting, horrible behavior were not dignified with the term "victim," since stalking was not a crime.

Many women fought long and hard to have their situations taken seriously and to be recognized as legitimate crime victims, so I use the term "stalking victim" here in honor of their legislative success.

❖ *Necessary and unnecessary fear*

Stalking victims are continuously confronted with the possibility of frightening, unpleasant actions against them, ranging from invasions of privacy all the way to lethal violence, but they are seldom given concrete, detailed advice on what to do about it. The purpose of this book is to change all that.

Some stalking victims are not as afraid as they should be, because they don't understand the seriousness of their situation. Other stalking victims are much more afraid than they need to be.

Many people are reluctant to label what they are experiencing as "stalking." This may reduce the amount of fear experienced, but it is just one more denial mechanism.

Security is like oxygen. When you have it, you never even give it a thought. When you don't have it, it is all you can think about!

Occasional fear is nature's way of making you pay attention to a dangerous situation, but constant, every day, extreme fear is not helpful. It is exhausting, debilitating, and soul-destroying. It is also unnecessary.

Unnecessary fear comes from not knowing what you would do if the situation you are in suddenly got worse. By being prepared and knowing what you would do in each situation, you can outwit your stalker, and keep your fear under control.

This book will show you how to learn to live in a state of "relaxed awareness." That may sound like a contradiction, but it is not.

❖ *Who stalks?*

Most stalkers, nearly 9 out or 10, are men. This is so overwhelmingly true that we will refer to stalkers in this book as "he," rather than as "he or she" (with apologies to the many good men who may be reading this).

Stalkers are very likely to be more intelligent than other criminals. They are also likely to be older than the average teen or twenty-something criminal; 35-40 years old is not unexpected, though they may range from youth to senior citizen. Stalkers come from all racial, ethnic, and socioeconomic groups.

Many of them have excellent manipulative skills that enable them to initiate contact with their victims without arousing suspicion.

Despite their intelligence, stalkers are very likely to be unemployed or under-employed. Some of them deliberately arrange their lives this way to allow plenty of time for their primary "occupation," stalking.

Many stalkers have some major stress in their lives a few weeks or months before they start stalking. The stress may be the loss of a job, the loss of a close relationship, financial pressure, illness, or even immigration to a new country.

Stalkers are likely to have some criminal behavior in their background, though they might never have been arrested for it. They may also have some psychiatric or substance abuse history.

Many stalkers, particularly those who are not the smooth, manipulative type, are socially incompetent, socially isolated loners who have great difficulty establishing and maintaining normal relationships. These stalkers may have a long history of failed relationships behind them. They may even have a history of stalking other people, sometimes many others.

A great many stalkers claim to be infatuated with their targets. As Linden Gross, author of a superb book on stalking and the creator of the Stalking Victim's Sanctuary website, explains, "The person with whom he's infatuated becomes his reason to exist. Any contact is better than no contact, any information a way to feel more intimately involved even if no relationship exists. That emptiness also helps explain the explosion that takes place during the separation or divorces of many couples, when those who have used their relationship to define their identity simply can't afford to let go."

While it is difficult to make generalizations about the personalities of stalkers, here are some characteristics that many stalkers seem to have in common:

- Won't take "no" for an answer
- Is jealous, possessive
- Has no close friends
- Is completely oblivious to logical arguments about his behavior
- Doesn't display the discomfort or anxiety that most people feel in certain situations (such as being caught in a lie)
- Tends to be obsessed with things (such as gambling) or people (such as entertainers)
- Has low self-esteem
- Lacks conscience; feels no remorse; doesn't see how his actions are hurting others
- Cannot learn from experience

- Believes society's rules don't apply to him
- Becomes violent when frustrated
- Is not capable of acting in his own self-interest.

It is also difficult to generalize about a stalker's motives. From the perspective of you, the recipient of the stalker's horrible behavior, it probably feels like your stalker is trying to control you, drive you crazy, upset your life, or make you extremely afraid.

From exhaustive interviews with stalkers, however, researchers have found a number of different motives from the stalkers' point of view. They include:

- Infatuation (seeking to establish or maintain a relationship)
- Delusion that the two of you have (or are destined to have) a relationship
- Identity-seeking (the stalker feels he needs you in his world or he will disappear)
- Possessiveness
- Anger
- Rejection (the stalker feels you rejected him)
- Retaliation for real or imagined wrongs

You may never know exactly what is motivating your stalker to behave the way he does. Fortunately, you don't need to know that in order to make yourself safe from whatever his plans are for you.

• **Are stalkers mentally ill?**

Mental disorders and personality disorders are fairly common among stalkers, though it would be incorrect to say that most stalkers are mentally ill.

It would also be incorrect to say that mentally ill people are likely to become stalkers.

Fortunately, stalkers are unlikely to be delusional or psychotic, though some few are.

Mental health professionals distinguish between major mental illnesses, such a schizophrenia or bipolar disorder, and severe personality disorders, which include borderline, narcissistic, antisocial, or dependent. You will probably not know whether your stalker falls into any of these groups, but if you do know his mental health history, it might help to explain some of his actions.

Psychotic stalkers, for example, are more likely to appear near your home, but are less likely to send letters. Non-psychotic stalkers make verbal threats more often, and are also more likely to become violent than psychotic stalkers.

Can counseling or other interventions stop a stalker? Again, there is no simple answer. Getting professional treatment for substance abuse problems or mental illness may help some stalkers change their behavior, but there is no simple cure.

One thing is clear. You, the victim, are never the appropriate person to try to administer counseling to the stalker. Leave that to the professionals.

❖ *Types of stalkers*

There is no single agreed-upon way to divide stalkers into categories, but we have merged several different approaches to stalker categorization into the following 4 sections: the stalker you know, the stalker you don't know, the stalker who thinks you love him (or her), and the "celebrity" stalker.

•   The stalker you know

You may know your stalker casually or have had a relationship with him in the past. He may be a former husband or boyfriend, whether there was domestic violence in the relationship or not. He may be someone you have rejected for a date, or someone you know casually from work, school, or other activities. He may even be a family member such as a brother, son, or father!

Just because you know him does not mean you did something to deserve this kind of treatment. Quite the contrary, because men with personalities that make them try to control women often have a charming social facade, so it is easy to be taken in by them at first. Don't berate yourself, thinking "I should have seen earlier that he was weird." He probably wasn't weird earlier, and there was nothing for you to pick up on. Concentrate instead on what you can do now.

The most common type of stalking situation, by far, is a man stalking a woman with whom he has been sexually intimate. If this is happening to you, you are definitely not alone. He may be trying to get you back, or he may be trying to intimidate and control you. Or both.

A person who has been excessively jealous and possessive in a relationship sometimes feels completely dependent on the person he purports to love, and can react with rage when the relationship is ending.

Closely related to this kind of stalker is one who has not been intimate with his target, but wants to be. He may be completely obsessed with you, or may be what one expert calls an "incompetent suitor," someone sincerely trying to establish a relationship, but who is completely lacking in courting skills. This kind of stalker may be supremely indifferent to the fact that you have repeatedly rejected him.

A completely different type of stalker is someone with whom you've never been intimate, but who had a grudge against you. It might be someone you know through work. Perhaps you are a boss or supervisor who had to give someone a bad review, or even terminate their employment. Now their resentment has taken the form of stalking and threats.

A resentful stalker usually feels oppressed by a whole series of imagined or actual incidents in which he felt powerless or humiliated, and he holds you responsible. You don't have to be the person involved in those incidents; some stalkers with a grudge against a particular company or organization will simply choose any accessible representative of that company to be the target of their attempts at revenge and retribution.

Campaign workers are another population from which stalkers can emerge. A number of state and national candidates have been stalked by people who originally got close to them by working on their campaign staffs.

Regardless of the type of prior relationship, stalkers who are motivated by resentment or the desire for revenge are often particularly persistent and intrusive.

Fortunately, your knowledge of the stalker can help you formulate your defenses against him!

• **The stalker you don't know**

Sometimes, stalkers pick targets that they have had no prior relationship with, or you may not yet have enough information to know for sure whether your stalker is a stranger to you or not.

In this case, you may begin to fear everyone, since your stalker may be, literally, anyone.

Although you may feel a strong desire, nearly a compulsion, to find out who he is, that should not be your top priority. It is much more important to keep yourself safe. In any choice between staying safe and learning his identity, choose safety!

Most likely, this type of stalker is someone who wants to pursue a relationship with you, but who is completely socially inept. He may prefer to admire you, and communicate with you, from afar, because he is afraid to actually be near you. If he communicates, it may be awkward, excessive, and just plain inappropriate.

It is very unlikely that your stalker is a predator whose primary intent is to rape or kill you (a type discussed more fully in the Celebrity Stalking section below), but since most predators are strangers to their targets, the possibility should be mentioned.

Not knowing who is pursuing you is particularly alarming and confusing, but you can take precautions to protect yourself from virtually all the things he might do, even if you never find out who he is, or why he chose you. This book will show you how.

•   The stalker who thinks you love him (or her)

There is a type of mental disorder called erotomania (pronounced er-rot-o-MANE-ee-a), in which the stalker has an absolutely unshakable belief, a delusion, actually, that his target is in love with him.

Or *she* has a delusion that her target is in love with *her*. This is the only type of stalking where the stalker is likely to be female. Often an erotomaniac stalker is a young woman who is obsessed with an older, higher-status man. She truly believes that he loves her, and that only circumstances, or perhaps other people, are keeping them apart from their mutual destiny.

This kind of stalker may believe that you are sending her communications that signal your love for her. Those "communications" of love may be the particular color of the coat you wore on a specific day, or the fact that you chatted with her about the weather at a bus stop, or they may be in her head entirely.

A well-known case of erotomaniac stalking is detailed in a book by Doreen Orion, a psychiatrist who was stalked for years by a woman who had, briefly, been a patient of hers.

Erotomaniac stalkers may have other significant mental illnesses, such as schizophrenia or bipolar (manic-depressive) disorder.

Erotomaniac stalking is quite rare, but tends to go on for a very long time, sometimes for many years.

• The celebrity stalker

You don't have to be a movie star or a famous singer to be targeted by a celebrity stalker. If you are in the public eye, if you appear on television or radio, if you are any kind of media reporter, if you have a high status professional job that brings you into contact with a large number of people, or if you are a public official, you may become the target of a celebrity stalker's attention. Doctors, lawyers, social workers, therapists, and teachers are just some of the professionals very much at risk for "celebrity" stalkers.

One expert source claims that radio personalities are at particularly high risk for stalking, since they often cultivate a personal, almost intimate relationship with their audience.

Another expert believes that female singers are at much higher risk than other kinds of performers, because their ability to communicate emotions through their music can make a stalker think the performance is just for him.

What everyone agrees on is that a "sexy" persona is *not* a magnet for stalkers. On the contrary, a wholesome, girl- or guy-next-door image is more receptive to the fantasies built by people whose social skills and self-image are seriously impaired. Gavin de Becker says, "The nicer one appears to be, and the more approachable, the more one will attract the serious and persistent and deluded subjects."

And of course, celebrities get their share of erotomanic stalkers, too, like Ralph Nau, who was absolutely convinced that Olivia Newton-John, Cher, and Sheena Easton had all proclaimed their love for him through hidden messages delivered during their TV shows.

Celebrity stalking is fairly rare. Even in Los Angeles, celebrity stalking is less than a third of the LA Police Department's Threat Management Unit's caseload. Most stalkers target ordinary people.

Celebrity stalkers are very different from domestic violence stalkers. Celebrity stalkers are seldom known to their victims before the stalking starts. They are likely to be socially incompetent, likely to have a mental illness, and often persist in their unwanted behavior for a longer time. They may stalk a famous person in order to gain fame that they cannot achieve any other way.

Your celebrity stalker may or may not want to get close to you physically. He may be so in awe of you that he can't imagine actually being in your presence. He may collect huge amounts of personal information about you, to give him a sense of intimacy without having to deal with actual interpersonal issues.

He is more likely to have an obvious mental disorder than most stalkers coming out of a domestic violence relationship, and he may think that he has a special, secret, mystical relationship with you.

Robert Bardo tried unsuccessfully to stalk several different celebrities in several different states, and finally fixated on 21-year-old television star Rebecca Schaeffer. He stalked her for months, finally located her home address, and shot her to death when she opened her door. Not all stories end so tragically.

A U.S. Border Patrol agent named Howard Schroeder stalked Holly Herbert, 31, a local TV news anchorwoman in Bakersville, CA, from January until May 1999. He wrote her letters and requested dates; she never responded in any way and never met him. When she got a restraining order against him, he had to turn over his weapons.

The good news here is that, although these stalkers may send endless communications such as cards and letters to you, or even approach your home, they often stop well short of face-to-face meetings. Threats, though they happen in a majority of cases, are rarely followed through.

The bad news here is that, if your stalker isn't one of the star-struck inept ones, he or she may be a truly dangerous predator, the kind who does not give warnings in the form of threats, but can be extremely dangerous, because they intend their victims great harm.

An example of such a predator is Jonathan Norman, who stalked the movie director Stephen Spielberg for a month, intending to rape Spielberg while forcing the director's wife to watch. He tried several times to break into Spielberg's estate, and when he was finally arrested, he was carrying a "rape kit" consisting of a knife, razor blades, handcuffs, and tape. He is now in prison, serving a 25-year sentence.

A predator like Norman carefully plans an attack, and uses stalking techniques to learn enough about his victim to organize the attack. These sorts of stalkers are the ones you meet most often in the movies, on the screen. Fortunately, they are extremely rare in real life. Nonetheless, because they don't give a lot of warning, it is important, and easier than you think, to protect against them.

The organization you work for may have resources to help protect you, particularly if the stalking is clearly related to your work, but even if that is not the case, this book will show you how to take better care of yourself.

❖ *"Why me?"*

Keep in mind that you are absolutely NOT to blame for what is happening. You do not "deserve" to be stalked—no matter what your stalker says!

You did absolutely nothing to "cause" his bad behavior.

Don't waste another minute asking yourself unanswerable "Why?" questions. Concentrate instead on asking "What" and "How" questions, like "What should I do to protect my unlisted phone number?" and "How can I safely get to work every day?" Answers to "what" and "how" questions can save your sanity, and also your life!

❖ *"It's not fair!"*

You are right, it is terribly unfair for you to have to go to the trouble of learning to stay safe. Real life isn't fair. Life is what it is, and you must make the best of your situation.

Yes, your stalker should be locked up, but he probably won't be anytime soon. Even if you do get him locked up, the moment he is out on bail or on parole, he may pick up right where he left off.

No, you cannot count on police, courts, restraining orders, employers, security personnel, or anyone else to protect you completely. You should, of course, take full advantage of all of those people and organizations as part of your personal protection plan, but they are only part of the plan, not all of it.

John Douglas, former chief of the FBI's Investigative Support Unit, and stalking expert, puts it quite directly: "For the victim to improve her situation, she must change her behavior."

The only way to feel better, and to be safer, is for you to *take control of your own safety*, and take positive steps to protect yourself!

❖ *"So, how much danger am I in?"*

If you are being stalked, you are afraid. Someone out there is targeting you. He is doing things that no rational person would do, and that scares you deeply. You keep wondering, "What is my stalker capable of?"

Even the non-violent stalker robs you of peace, privacy, and happiness. **Around one third of stalkers become violent.** Some of that violence is directed against property, some of it is directed against the stalker's victim, and some of it may be directed against other people.

Rhonda Saunders, the prosecutor who put many stalkers, including Madonna's, in prison, thinks the homicide rate of stalking victims might be as high as the 2-5% range. Another stalking expert has estimated that around 1-2% of stalking victims are murdered. A more recent estimate puts it well under 1%.

Does that number make you feel safe ("Wow, 99% of stalking victims aren't killed!"), or does it make you worry more? After all, far fewer than 1% of police or taxi drivers are killed on the job, so even this low murder rate puts you in more danger than if you were a member of those notoriously "high risk" professions! That's why it is so important to take safety precautions that may seem extreme to people who are not at risk.

The bottom line: It is impossible to predict exactly which stalkers will be violent, and when.

Every case is different, but, if you know your stalker and, based on his prior actions with you, you think you are in danger from him, you probably are! If you don't know your stalker, but his actions are frightening you, don't ignore your fear!

All stalking victims should get some help evaluating their level of peril! The organizations listed in the appendices can help you find people to do this kind of evaluation.

Evaluating dangerousness is a very inexact science. There is no such thing as a simple checklist that will determine how violence-prone a stalker is or whether an attack is likely. That said, here are some generalities that should be used with extreme care:

- Fewer than half of stalkers make overt threats, but the ones who don't threaten can be just as dangerous as those who do threaten.
- If your stalker is a former sexual partner, particularly if there is a history of violence between you, your danger is increased.
- If your stalker is a resentful ex-employee, you are probably in less physical danger than you would be from an ex-intimate partner. Resentment seems to incite harassment, but it seldom turns into assault.
- If you are a "celebrity" being stalked by someone, even someone with a mental disorder, you aren't necessarily in a lot of danger, though such stalkers may become frustrated, angry, and even violent when they finally realize that their affection for you is not returned.
- If you have an stalker who thinks you are in love with her (or him), you probably are not in a lot of danger yourself, but the stalker may go after anyone who she thinks is coming between the two of you.
- Stalkers who think you rejected them, and stalkers whose sense of identity is completely dependent on you, are among the most likely to use intimidation as a tactic, and to become violent.
- Stalkers who have a history of violence (including access to guns) are more likely to be violent than those who don't have those interests.
- Stalkers who abuse alcohol or drugs are more dangerous than those who don't.
- Female stalkers are less dangerous than male stalkers.

- Stalkers with severe personality disorders are more dangerous than those without these mental problems.
- Stalkers who are unemployed or socially isolated are more likely to be violent than those who are employed and have a network of social connections.
- If your stalker is extremely angry at you, that raises your level of danger.
- If you don't take enough extra safety precautions, your increase the amount of danger you are in.

You must treat your stalker as if he or she is extremely dangerous, and stay away from the stalker as completely as possible.

Your stalker's behavior cannot be predicted precisely, and it can change very, very quickly. You have to be ready for anything.

It is hard for women to "be ready for anything" since they aren't usually given much detailed, concrete advice on how to be ready or what to do if "anything" happens. The purpose of this book to change all that, starting with the notion of relaxed awareness.

❖ *Relaxed awareness*

Although most stalking situations last a year or less, many are longer, and a few last for decades! Some stalkers continue stalking as soon as they finish a prison term for stalking.

Rhonda Saunders, the Assistant District Attorney who successfully prosecuted many stalkers, says, "Stalking cases never end."

This means that once you become the target of a stalker, stalking will be a major part of your life for a long time. That's a strong motivation to make permanent changes in your lifestyle to ensure your safety. There are no quick fixes to being stalked. So how can you deal with such a stressful crime that may go on for years?

A favorite quotation from James Thurber says a lot: "Do not look back in anger, or forward in fear, but around in awareness."

Many folks experienced in self protection use a system of levels of awareness to help themselves understand and change their awareness. Here is a quick introduction to the levels of awareness:

Unaware. This is the state you are in when you are virtually unaware of who and what is around you. In this condition, you are easily startled, because you are surprised by anyone who is near you. Folks in this condition walk around with their eyes on the ground, their ears covered with earphones, and their minds a million miles away. They work totally engrossed at their computer screens, with their backs to the office door, oblivious of who might be there. They sit "spaced out" in their cars in traffic.

You have probably lived most of your life in this state, but it isn't very safe, because you are vulnerable when you aren't aware of what is going on around you. By being totally unaware, you look and act like a victim—if your stalker doesn't get you, maybe a mugger will!

Relaxed Awareness. In this state of awareness, you are conscious of who is around you, what vehicles are nearby, what escape routes you might use if necessary, and so on.

You will not be startled by the sudden presence of another person, because you already know who is there. Folks in this condition walk around with their heads up and their eyes level, and simply notice their environment. Their manner is relaxed, but not sloppy.

Just as you can drive competently and vigilantly while simultaneously carrying on a conversation, you can learn to carry on your normal activities while simultaneously adding an awareness of your surroundings.

Well-trained police officers are in this condition whenever they are on the job, and the best ones maintain that level of awareness in their private lives. People who are being stalked should be in this condition nearly all of their waking hours.

This level of awareness, of just noticing what is going on around you, is not stressful; once you are accustomed to it, you can maintain it for months or years without ill effect!

Active Concern. This is the state when something out of the ordinary has happened to catch your attention. That something represents a potential threat, but is not an actual threat yet.

Perhaps you notice the same car driving behind you for a long time. Perhaps you hear a noise outside your home at night. Perhaps you see a person approaching you who does not seem to be acting normally. These are potential problems, not direct attacks on you.

In this level, you should be consciously evaluating the dangerousness of your situation and your options for action. "What are the places I could drive to if that car keeps following me?" "Which telephone will I use, if that noise outside is someone trying to get in?" "What are the things I could do or say if that man approaches me?"

You may have to remind yourself to breathe, because we all naturally tend to hold our breath when anxious or surprised. But consciously forcing yourself to take a few deep breaths will help you get ready to react, and will remind you that YOU are in control, not the person who is alarming you.

Because you are, naturally, afraid, this level of awareness is stressful, and cannot be maintained indefinitely. However, it is OK to be in this state for many minutes, many times a day, as long as you have periods of relaxed awareness in between.

Extreme Danger! This is the condition we would all like to avoid, the situation of being attacked by another person.

In this level, you know exactly who the threat is and what he is trying to do. You will be very afraid. You will react as you have been trained, or as you planned to do when you were merely actively concerned. This book will help you train and plan for such a situation. You must put your plan into action to protect yourself. Depending on the circumstances, your plan may be to run, to hide, or to fight; whatever it is, do it immediately!

Stalking and Awareness

So, how do all these conditions relate to stalking? Most people have no self-defense training, or no training relevant to the situation they find themselves in when they are being stalked. They bounce wildly from being completely unaware to near panic whenever their stalker makes a move, even if they just think there might be a problem. They constantly live in fear, in the highest two levels of readiness, and that unceasing stress takes a terrible toll over time.

Remember, "necessary fear" is what you feel when someone has actually threatened you, invaded your home, or done something else to put you in immediate danger. "Unnecessary fear" is feeling that same high level of fright when you are at home alone, or any other time that you are not really in danger, but you feel afraid anyway.

This book will show you how to remove unnecessary fear from your life, and replace it with relaxed awareness.

2 The First, Most Essential Things To Do

It would be wonderful if you could simply tell the police, your employer, or your family about your problem, and let them handle the whole situation. But that's a dream, not real life.

Many of the measures necessary for protection against stalking must be taken by you, the victim. Fortunately, you are NOT defenseless!!

❖ *Take responsibility for your own safety*

Nobody else can do as good a job of protecting you as you can. You are the only person who is with you 24 hours a day, 7 days a week, 52 weeks a year. You know your lifestyle, your needs, and your circumstances. You don't yet fully understand or appreciate your defensive capabilities, but you will learn, and then you will become confident in your ability to triumph over your stalker.

As the ongoing victim of an ongoing crime, you are in the best position to take responsibility for your own safety.

Taking responsibility for your own safety means that you should:

✓   Know your situation, and what you can realistically do.
✓   Learn new skills and techniques to deal with the stalking, both as it is now and as it may develop.

✓ Understand what other people might do to help keep you safe and stop the stalker.

✓ Learn how to live a reasonably normal life, safely, without unnecessary fear.

Taking responsibility for your own safety does NOT mean:

✗ Having a false sense of security.

✗ Being "paranoid," hypervigilant, barricaded in your home, running scared, or afraid to go out.

✗ That your life will be exactly as it was before the stalking started.

✗ That you alone have to do everything necessary to assure your safety.

The police can help a lot, but do not expect the police to protect you, or to even take the lead in gathering evidence, capturing and incarcerating your stalker. You will probably have to do a lot of work on your own case.

A police officer in the Los Angeles Police Department's Threat Management Unit said "We treat victims as clients. This is their problem. They will get help in managing their problem. But it's unrealistic to expect that life will improve just by filing a police report."

Put another way, "The stalking problem belongs to the victim…all these different agencies…are there to help that person manage the problem, but it's their problem."

An article by Ellen Sorokin in the Washington Times confirms this. She says, "The laws rarely work. If you believe in them too much, they can get you hurt."

This is a bitter pill to swallow. We would all like to believe that when we are in trouble, when we are the victim of a serious crime that may put us in extraordinary danger, the police will spring into action to protect us. We expect relief from the fear, and it hurts terribly to get the message, "There's not much we can do."

Fortunately, that message will be heard less and less often as police and prosecutors and the criminal justice system learn how to handle the crime of stalking. However, even the best police units in the world, such as the Los Angeles stalking unit, know that they cannot protect any stalking victim every day and every night for as long as it takes to get the stalker off the streets.

You have to learn to protect yourself. And you can!!

❖ *"He's trying to drive me crazy, and I'm not going to give him the satisfaction!"*

Is that how you feel? If so, you probably know who your "enemy" is. You two probably know one another very well, and he knows how to push all your buttons.

Naturally, you are angry. You want to get even. You want him to stop his childish, immature (but incredibly annoying) harassment. You also want him to acknowledge that what he has been doing is wrong.

You don't want to have to change yourself.

It is a battle of wills, and you want to crow over every point you score.

This book isn't going to have much of interest for you. Why not? Because you still have a relationship with him, even if it is based on anger. You are continuing to engage in the back-and-forth of that relationship, rather than break it off completely and finally.

You are choosing the relationship over your own safety.

Every woman in the world can relate to this, because we've all been there. However, if this guy suddenly becomes dangerous, instead of merely annoying, you won't be ready for him.

If you really want the relationship, or are ambivalent about it, get some counseling to help you through this difficult time. If you really don't want the relationship, end it completely, and take some of the precautions in this book in case he doesn't take well to the ending.

❖ *"I'm not going to give in to my fear!"*

Let's talk about this "giving in to fear" thing. What does that mean to you? Would you be "giving in to fear" if you boldly took self defense courses, got better locks on your doors, got an unlisted phone number, and told your friends about the stalking that is going on in your life? Or would you be giving in to fear if you sat at home night after night, too terrified to go shopping or to the movies?

If you answered yes to the first question then, to you, not giving in to fear probably means making hardly any changes in your life, trying to live life "as usual."

There are lots of variations on this theme. When urged to take safety precautions, some people say, "I'm not going to do that because it would be giving the stalker power over me" or "I'm not going to take extreme precautions because I don't want to let the stalker affect my life that much."

The Anti-Stalking website (see Appendix A) says it best: "Stalking victims…will say, 'I won't let myself be victimized,' or 'I'm not going to change my life because I'm being stalked.' Sorry. Your life has changed. Forever. And unless you accept that, you will actually be helping the stalker."

That's right. By doing nothing differently, or not much, you help the stalker. It helps him to know your address, your phone number, and lots of details about your life. It helps him to know that, since you aren't enlisting any people to help you, he can continue to harass you without fear of anybody else's reaction. It helps him to know that you are just as defenseless now, as you were when he started his campaign of terror.

The stalker is like a critical illness in your life. If you do nothing but carry on your life "as usual," the result is going to be much more serious, perhaps deadly, than if you had sought help early. The help for an illness is getting involved in medical treatment; the help for stalking is getting involved in your own safety.

Don't let them call you paranoid. When an arsonist threatens your home, or when the nearest fire station is miles away, it is prudent, not paranoid, to buy a couple of fire extinguishers. When you have a stalker in your life, it is prudent, not paranoid, to take safety precautions that others might find extreme.

Good advice that people often get is "Don't let him see how scared you are." But how can you carry it out when you are terrified by every move he makes? Some women just try to live "as usual" without changing anything about their activities, thinking that this will send an "I'm not scared" message to their tormentor. Wrong. It lets him see your reaction to the things he says and does, which is exactly what he wants, and it does nothing to keep you safe. So, how can you keep him from seeing your reactions to his frightening activities?

Fortunately, most of the suggestions in this book will increase your safety while being invisible to him, or at least not giving him the chance to see how he is affecting you. All he will know is that he can't reach you on the phone any more, can't find your car to follow home after work any more, can't see you through your windows at night, and can't even tell for sure whether you have changed jobs or moved. He will be unable to determine whether you are still afraid of him, or just indifferent to him.

Meantime, your new safety-conscious habits and air of relaxed awareness will be keeping you safe, and making you less afraid.

❖ *How to prevent stalking from starting*

For most of us, the best way to avoid ever becoming a stalker's target is to avoid, or immediately get out of, a relationship with anyone whose personality or history shows the warning signs of violence, excessive jealousy, substance abuse, extreme dependency, or wild mood swings.

For professional people, managers, media figures, political figures, and others who might become the target of a "celebrity" stalker, there are more steps that can easily be taken:

Get an unlisted phone number and a private mail box. Follow the suggestions in Chapter 3 on safeguarding your personal information. Consider using a pseudonym, particularly if you have an on-air media job.

As a potential celebrity stalking target, you have two goals, one is to keep away from the wierd-but-probably-harmelss people who may harass you. The other goal is to keep away from the predators, the stalkers who, though few in number, silently stalk their victims while plotting serious attacks, usually of a sexual nature.

The security organization of the place where you work can definitely help with the first kind of stalker. You should be sure that they have procedures in place, for example, so that a "fan" who shows up looking for you will not be able to see you in person, and will not be told any non-public information about you ("She usually leaves here around 3 P.M."). Also security personnel should intercept and check any packages and gifts that are delivered.

A predatory stalker won't show up with a strange letter for you, however. He is much more likely to watch you from a distance, find out where you live, and follow you to determine your daily schedule. All of the steps in this book to safeguard your home address and phone will be useful against this type of stalker, as will awareness on your part of whether someone is following you; there is plenty of advice in this book on how to determine that, and what to do about it.

❖ *As soon as you* think *you might have a problem*

At this point, someone or something is making you nervous. You might or might not be able to explain it to someone else. You wonder, "How seriously should I take this?"

Don't ignore it, or try to minimize it. The proper actions taken at this time may discourage your harasser, and keep him from turning into a full-fledged stalker.

What should you do if the guy you dated a few times and are no longer interested in keeps calling? What should you do if a guy you don't want to go out with keeps pestering you for a date? What should you do if you start getting amorous, inappropriate, anonymous email that makes you cringe? What should you do if you don't know whether the guy is just persistent, or a bit weird? What should you do if you just don't know for sure that you have a problem on your hands?

• Be firm

If this is someone you have been dating, you may have to be very firm in breaking off the relationship. Don't try to let him down easily, for example by saying, "You're a great guy and you have a lot to offer, but I'm not the girl for you." He can interpret this as meaning that you like him, but that you are confused, and so he will continue to try to prove that you ARE the girl for him.

Here's Gavin de Becker's example of a firm, unconditional rejection: "No matter what you've assumed up to now, and no matter for what reason you assumed it, I have no romantic interest in you whatsoever. I am certain I never will. I expect that, knowing this, you will put your attention elsewhere, which I understand, because that's what I intend to do."

Even if it is not a dating relationship, you should be equally clear and firm when telling him to stop the behavior that is annoying you.

•   Be aware

Keep your eyes and ears open. You don't want to miss any signals about your problem. You do not need to take any extreme steps for your safety at this stage, but you should take increased precautions.

If you get odd letters, presents, or other communications, keep them. If you get the feeling that someone is following you, look around and see.

Mention to your friends and family what is happening that makes you suspicious or concerned. This allows them to be alert for any unusual circumstances, too.

•   Think ahead

This is a good time to review your basic safety precautions, and to look through the rest of this book for a few new ones to add to your daily routine.

Start thinking about alternatives. "If he calls more frequently than twice a day, I'll report him to the police." "I'll check my rear view mirror more often, so he can't follow me home."

Planning ahead **always** gives you the edge over your antagonist.

❖ *As soon as you* know *you have a problem*

At this point, you are feeling scared. Don't ignore it, or try to minimize it. He won't "just go away." You need to start taking some very active measures.

• **Have NO contact**

> The most important thing you can do to ensure your safety and to minimize the stalker's impact on your life is to completely avoid ALL contact with him.

That's the most important sentence in this whole book!

Every time your stalker gets to see you, to talk to you, to learn some personal information about you, to hear your voice, to peer in your windows or stand in your home, he feels rewarded for his efforts in pursuing you.

If he has to call you 50 times before you pick up the phone and yell at him, he has just learned to make 50, or 60, or 100 calls next time before you reward him by answering the phone.

One reason for the firm "no contact" rule is to avoid rewarding his behavior. Another reason for it is to protect you in case he is becoming violent.

Robert Snow, a police captain who has written extensively on stalking, says, "If the victims can successfully isolate themselves from their stalkers, the ability of the stalkers to intimidate them becomes negligible and the stalking a failure."

Gavin de Becker, one of the world's experts on this crime, advocates a policy of "aggressive nonintervention." In one unambiguous communication, he says, quickly and firmly break all contact with the perpetrator, including all indirect contact by friends, family, police, or restraining orders. Then watch the stalker's actions. There may be a period of continued contact, or even an escalation of stalking behaviors. The stalking victim must have tremendous patience, strength, and courage during this time to maintain the "detach and watch strategy," but it is often very effective.

Keeping the no contact rule can be quite hard, particularly if your stalker is your ex-husband and you have children together. How can you have no, or minimal contact with someone when you have to share custody or at least arrange the kids' visits and hand them back and forth? We provide some detailed suggestions in a later section.

The rest of this book has a large number of very concrete suggestions about how to maintain "no contact" at home, at work, or in public, how to keep him from finding out the information he needs to pursue you (such as your phone number and where you live), and how to be prepared for anything he might do.

• Keep good records

The next most important thing is to keep accurate, complete records of all stalking behavior, including evidence that may be useful in court.

This log can be critical in convincing police, juries, judges, and parole officers that this man is a threat. Doreen Orion, a psychiatrist who was stalked for many years, took shopping bags full of her logs and notes to various court appearances; her stalker eventually served time for violating restraining orders.

Even if your stalker is never arrested and tried, the log will give you a sense of control over the situation, and it will help you prove to other people what you have been going through.

Write down every time you think the stalker calls you, details of every time he tries to contact you, and any gifts he leaves or sends to you. Record the day, time, location, and what happened. If there were witnesses around, record their names, too. Try to write precisely what the stalker said and did, and what you said and did.

Keep a copy in a safe place, in case he manages to steal the original. Appendix B has a sample stalking log format.

To supplement your written records, keep a camera handy, either the point-and-shoot variety or a video camera. Do not try to take photos of your stalker—that is much too dangerous! The camera is to take pictures of any vandalism you think he is responsible for, and any perishable things he sends you, such as flowers, food, and candy.

Some cameras can date and time stamp the photos automatically; if yours does not have this feature, have the film developed as soon as possible, and put the date the photo was taken on the back of each one. Keep the dated photos with explanatory notes as part of your log.

When the stalker sends you things that are not perishable, handle them as little as possible, and put them in clear plastic bags marked with the date to preserve them to use as evidence. Always keep the envelopes and wrapping materials as well as the contents.

Keep all the evidence in a very safe place.

• Don't try to reason with him—he's not rational

You must realize that your stalker is, more likely than not, NOT a rational human being. Trying to anticipate the motives, agenda or moves of a person who is thinking irrationally is virtually impossible for a normal human being to do.

One stalking victim says, "I made this mistake on countless occasions and I remember saying to myself over and over again, in total disbelief, 'I never thought he could do that.' Well, the truth of the matter is that it is almost impossible to have the insight into the irrational mind to glean a hint of what is possible, if you are not a psych professional or irrational yourself.

Once I learned this, but more importantly, once I believed it, I was better able to make safer decisions for myself."

> Reasoning with him is not an option because it is impossible to reason with an irrational mind. This is many stalking victims' biggest and worst mistake.

The same stalking victim goes on, "Women tend to think that we have the ability to change men, even psychotic ones, by communicating or reasoning with them. Wrong! Never!! Ever!!! "

Irrationality isn't always blatant. He may appear concerned, kind, and dedicated to "working things out" with you. Don't fall for it. His persistence and inability to hear you say "no" will give him away.

• Learn the law

The law is powerful, and anti-stalking laws are in effect in every state. But laws vary by location, and can change quickly. Check with local women's shelters, a local lawyer, a prosecutor, or your state Attorney General to find out exactly what the current laws relevant to stalking are in your area.

Important legal concepts also differ from place to place, for example:

What, exactly, constitutes stalking?

Does the stalker have to make a threat? What is a threat, or a credible threat? Do actions ever constitute a threat, or must it be words?

Who is your "immediate family"; does this include unrelated people in your household?

What constitutes a course of conduct—2 instances? 3? 10? Over what period of time—1 hour? 1 day? more than 1 week?

In some locales, police can arrest a stalker in misdemeanor cases, even if they do not witness the crime; in other places, they must see the crime.

In some places, prosecutors pursue most stalking cases; in other places, hardly any. Depending on the law, and the particular people charged with enforcing it, stalking might be easy to prove, or more difficult to prove than murder.

There is a federal law called the Interstate Stalking Punishment and Prevention Act. This law makes it a federal crime, punishable by up to 5 years in prison, to cross state lines to stalk someone. It is difficult, but not impossible, to have a stalker prosecuted under this law.

Understanding exactly what is and isn't stalking where you live will help you know what behaviors to watch for, and will make it easier if you try to get your stalker arrested. If what he is doing does not fit your local stalking statute, perhaps other charges can be brought against him.

Much legal information is available on the Internet; see the listings in Appendix A for some good starting points.

❖ *Take control*

Schaum and Parrish say, "The sense of purpose and power in taking action, uniting with others to provide personal support and fight back…, can be invaluable ways of reclaiming control."

Taking back a sense of control over your life consists of 3 steps: appraising your situation realistically, making a safety plan, and working with others to carry it out.

• Appraise your situation

Understand everything you can about your situation.

This means learning everything you can about stalking from books, organizations, web sites, and community resources. The lists in the appendices of this book are a good starting point.

Learn as much as you can about your stalker, without endangering yourself.

Talk with experts who can help you assess the level of danger that you are in. Again, the appendices provide a lot of starting points.

• Decide on a strategy

There are two primary strategies to managing a stalking situation. You can only pick one of them at a time, so you may want to read the rest of this book before you decide between them.

The first strategy is called Intervention. Its purpose is to try to make the stalker modify his behavior. It generally involves communicating to the stalker your absolute non-interest in him. This message can be delivered in person, through police or other security-oriented personnel, or via a restraining order, but it must be a strong, unequivocal message. Then, if the stalker ignores your warning or violates the restraining order, you try to bring the strongest possible consequences to bear on him.

The advantages of this strategy is that it usually involves societal pressure, not just your own actions. The disadvantage is that sometimes the legal sanctions that ought to be there aren't strong enough, or don't happen at all, sending your stalker the message that there will be no negative consequences for his acts.

The second strategy is called Non-Intervention. Its purpose is to keep you out of contact with the stalker, not to change his behavior. This may also involve a single unequivocal statement to the stalker that you are not interested in his attentions, but that statement comes from you. Then, you do nothing except break off absolutely every bit of contact with the stalker. You never let him hear your voice, or see you, or learn any more than he already knows about you. You don't send any indirect messages via the police or other people. You don't get a restraining order. You simply insulate yourself from him as completely as possible, then wait him out. It is difficult, but a great many stalkers will give up (and possibly move on to some other target).

The advantage of the non-intervention strategy is that it is almost completely under your own control. The disadvantage is that you do not have as much involvement of police or the courts at an early stage of the stalking, though of course you can always switch to an intervention strategy later if the situation demands it.

With either strategy, you should take a lot of steps to protect yourself from your stalker, and this book will show you how. In Chapter 13 there is a discussion of the pros and cons of restraining orders, to help you decide which strategy to pursue.

• Make a safety plan

Make a clear, objective, reasonable plan of action to maximize your safety.

Some parts of the plan may be things you can do immediately, such as talking to the police. Some parts might be longer range, such as taking a series of self-defense courses.

This book has a lot of suggestions to help you develop such a plan.

• Work with others

Isn't it good news that you don't have to do it all alone?

Let other people help to achieve your plan.

Tell the police. More victims are helped by law enforcement than are harmed, so definitely report your situation to the police, but try to be realistic in your expectations of what they can do.

Also tell your family, friends, co-workers, neighbors, and others you can trust exactly what is going on. If possible, give them a description of your stalker, or even a photograph, and any other information that will help them recognize him. Enlist their help as extra eyes and ears. Have them keep records of what they see and hear, to add to your own.

For women especiallyt, heightened safety lies in the details of the little everyday activities of life. Carrying out your safety plan must include attention to a lot of details at first, but those details will quickly become habits you don't even give much thought to.

Now let's get to some more very concrete things you can put in your safety plan, and ways for you to take action, reclaim control, and fight back effectively!!

3 Your Personal Information—A Stalker's Treasure

Your stalker's obsession may be to collect personal, even intimate information about you. This gives him a kick, a sense of being close to you. It probably bothers you to think he might be filling his room with papers pulled out of your trash. It will certainly bother you if he sends you letters filled with personal information about you that he has no right to know.

Perhaps your stalker's obsession is to find out where you live, and to get physically close to you. Almost every stalking victim has a deep fear of her stalker invading her home. How can you keep a stalker from finding out where you live, or what your phone number is?

The first step is to understand what and where your "personal information" is, and then you can learn how to safeguard it.

Remember, you do not have to do all of these things, just pick what is most relevant to you right now.

❖ Who has personal information about you?

This section lists some of the people and organizations that may have your name, address, various ID numbers, or other personal information. You can probably think of even more.

Personal Data
Personal papers
Services you have used in or near your home
Utility companies
Financial and medical institutions
Work-, home-, or school-related information
Phone-related organizations
Courts; criminal justice system
Companies
Federal, state, or local government

You might use the following list as a starting point to contact these people and organizations and explain that on principle you do not want to let your home address be known, so please will they change their records to your post office box or private mailbox address.

Another way to use this list is to contact the people on it who you consider most trustworthy, tell them that you are being stalked, and ask them to be particularly careful not to give out information about you to anyone on any pretext.

If these people and organizations don't already have information about you, you might want to be careful in the future not to give them any information you would not want a stalker to have!

Where is Your Personal Information?

➤ **Personal papers you have in your wallet, car, purse, or home**

✦ checks
✦ insurance cards
✦ "in case of emergency" card
✦ daily planner
✦ calendar
✦ address book
✦ photos of family members
✦ personal digital assistant (PDA)

➤ **Services you have used in or near your home**

✦ moving company
✦ plumber
✦ electrician
✦ pool cleaner
✦ chimney sweep
✦ yard work
✦ appliance repair
✦ snow shoveling or removal
✦ painting (interior, exterior)
✦ recycling or trash pickup
✦ food store
✦ car repair
✦ travel agent

✦ delivery services, such as pizza, newspapers, florists, groceries, etc.
✦ contractors of all kinds
✦ dry cleaner
✦ convenience stores
✦ check cashing services
✦ Mary Kay, Fuller Brush, Amway or Avon salespeople
✦ discount shopping clubs and stores
✦ "Frequent Flyer" or other such clubs and plans
✦ companies you rent things from. such as videos, cars, tools, and apartments
✦ magazine subscriptions
✦ newspaper subscriptions
✦ fitness or sports clubs
✦ hobby clubs, for quilting, books, coupons, fan clubs, shopping, and so on
✦ sports leagues
✦ organizations, schools, groups, or clubs your children are associated with
✦ veterinarian
✦ lawyers, both business and personal
✦ dating services

➤ **Utility companies**
✦ electric
✦ gas
✦ oil
✦ local telephone
✦ long distance telephone
✦ mobile telephone

- ❖ cable TV
- ❖ Internet service provider

➤ **Financial and medical institutions** (not just your own, but your children, spouse, and other family members)
- ❖ hospitals
- ❖ HMOs
- ❖ doctors' offices
- ❖ dentist's offices
- ❖ counselor, psychologist, psychiatrist
- ❖ social workers
- ❖ support groups
- ❖ clinics
- ❖ nursing homes or similar facilities
- ❖ pharmacies
- ❖ insurance companies for your home, car, business, medical, life
- ❖ medical information bureaus
- ❖ stores where you have a credit account
- ❖ credit card companies
- ❖ credit bureaus
- ❖ banks where you have accounts, loans, a safe deposit box, or other services
- ❖ any person or organization that has provided a loan
- ❖ financial planner
- ❖ tax advisor
- ❖ broker
- ❖ investment houses
- ❖ landlord's rental applications

✦   mortgage holders
✦   homeowners' or tenants" association

➤ Work-related

✦   company personnel records
✦   union records
✦   professional associations
✦   any organization that you have received any kind of training and certification or license from
✦   co-workers
✦   informal company publications such as newsletters, employee phone book, intranet, group address lists, club distribution lists
✦   co-workers' Rolodexes and personal phone records
✦   medical boards
✦   bar associations
✦   worker's compensation records
✦   email distribution lists
✦   work computer(s)
✦   online employee records

➤ Home- and school-related

✦   luggage tags
✦   return address stickers for envelopes
✦   backpacks
✦   neighbors
✦   friends
✦   family members
✦   any school you, your spouse, or your children have ever attended
✦   classmates

- ✦ teachers
- ✦ other school employees
- ✦ school "telephone tree" lists
- ✦ your children's friends and their families
- ✦ any person or organization that has provided a scholarship, counseling, tutoring, or other services
- ✦ college, junior college, or community college alumni offices
- ✦ any group that you have taken classes from. such as community adult education, museum schools, and job training

➤ Phone-related organizations

- ✦ any person or company you call on a toll free number. This includes the area codes 800, 900, 877, 888, and possibly others.
- ✦ "reverse phone directories" where you start with a phone number, look it up, and get the name and/or address of the person who has that phone. Unlisted numbers are not necessarily protected from these directories.
- ✦ companies providing paging services

➤ Courts and the criminal justice system

- ✦ courts where you have divorce records or child custody or support agreements
- ✦ courts where you have applied for a restraining order
- ✦ courts where you have sued someone, or have been sued
- ✦ victim witness advocates, social workers, or similar people associated with the court system
- ✦ local, state, or federal criminal justice system, if you have been involved there

- ✦ lawyers
- ✦ legal aid workers

➤ Companies and other organizations

- ✦ direct mail retailers. This is any company that sends you a catalog, whether you have purchased from them or not.
- ✦ Internet records, such as email, newsgroups, chat rooms, web sites, anyone who has your email address
- ✦ companies whose Internet website you have registered with, whether or not you have ordered products from them
- ✦ any company you have registered a product with, including computer software or hardware
- ✦ community organizations
- ✦ churches, mosques, synagogues and other religious organizations
- ✦ informal church publications such as newsletters and members' address lists
- ✦ newspaper archives, if you have ever been in the news
- ✦ charities or causes you have donated to
- ✦ political organizations you have donated to
- ✦ any organization that sends you requests for donations, whether you have contributed or not.
- ✦ public libraries
- ✦ hotels where you have stayed

➤ Federal government

- ✦ IRS
- ✦ Social Security Administration
- ✦ Veteran's Administration
- ✦ US Passport Agency

- ✦ Army, Navy, Air Force, Marine Corps, or Cost Guard
- ✦ any branch of the Reserves
- ✦ organizations of former military personnel
- ✦ Peace Corps
- ✦ US Civil Service
- ✦ any federal courts you have had dealings with

➤ State government
- ✦ state income or other tax records
- ✦ drivers license
- ✦ car registration
- ✦ car title
- ✦ welfare or food stamp records
- ✦ firearms licenses
- ✦ fishing or hunting licenses
- ✦ bankruptcy records
- ✦ abandoned property records
- ✦ any state certifications or licenses you hold, such as notary, CPA, building contractor, stock broker, pharmacist, therapist, teacher, beautician, barber, security guard, pilot, x-ray technician, real estate agent, and so on.

➤ Local (county, city) government
- ✦ Some local governments issue certifications or licenses such as those listed in the state government section
- ✦ property transfers and tax records
- ✦ excise tax
- ✦ water and sewer departments
- ✦ marriage license

❖   dog licenses
❖   local business licenses
❖   trust agreement
❖   boat registration
❖   voter registration
❖   divorce, separation and support agreements
❖   power of attorney
❖   jury duty lists
❖   change of name records
❖   birth records
❖   adoption records
❖   guardianship records
❖   foster care records
❖   deeds
❖   assignment of a lien or mortgage
❖   local police

❖ *"I know where you live!"—your address*

For most of us, our home is a sanctuary, the one place we can feel perfectly relaxed, comfortable, and safe. Keeping your stalker away from your home will give you much peace of mind, but you have to do some work to make this happen.

The two main issues of this section are how to keep the stalker from finding out your home address, and how to avoid using a mailbox that the stalker can easily steal from. (Yes, it is a federal crime to open someone else's mailbox and remove the contents, but when was the last time you heard about a prosecution for that crime?)

Protect Your Home Address
Don't give out your home address
Use a shredder
Change government records
Get a private mailbox or PO box
Use a mail drop
Remove information from credit agencies
Don't use a return address
Don't use your name
Have friends and family protect it, too

• Don't give out your address

The most basic rule is: Don't give your residential address to any person or organization. Use a post office box address, your work address, or your lawyer's address…anything but your true residence.

Do not put your residential address on any piece of paper you carry in your purse or wallet. Use a post office box address, or just leave it blank.

If someone insists on having your address, give them, without comment, the address of your attorney. This is particularly important if you must, by law, give them your real name instead of your alias, such as when you are making a financial transaction, real estate transaction, putting your name on a public record for voter registration or a library card, etc.

Consider using your lawyer's address for all important mail and notifications.

If you are lucky enough to live in California, and unlucky enough to be relocating because of domestic violence, you may be eligible for California's new "Safe at Home" program, which provides qualified people who need privacy with a substitute mailing address for use on all public records and documents. Mail sent to that address is then forwarded to the women within 2 days. By the time this book is in print, the protection may have been extended to stalking victims. Other states may develop similar programs; check with your Secretary of State's office.

•   Use a shredder

Inexpensive paper shredders are available at stores like Office Max and Staples. Shred ALL paper trash, especially anything with your name, address, credit card numbers, or other ID numbers. Assume that if the stalker hasn't already stolen and gone through your trash, he will! Remember, you have complete control over what goes into your trash.

•   Change government records

Get your address and other personal information removed from ALL government records. This is hard, because you will need to deal with each one separately. Review the beginning of this chapter for a list of government records that you may want to have changed

• **Private mailboxes, PO boxes**

A PRIVATE mailbox (PMB) such as MailBoxes Etc., Pony Express, or other services, is usually preferable to a US Post Office Box. Ideally, the mailbox should be some distance away from your home. Always give this mailbox as your "home address." Use this address on your driver's license, your car registration, and your checks.

All bills, newspapers, packages, and magazine subscriptions should go to the private mailbox, NOT to your true home address. The ONLY mail you should receive at home are personal letters from people you trust absolutely.

Do not let friends or relatives get magazine subscriptions for you with your true home address or send anything mail-order directly to your home.

If some organization wants your address, and says they will not accept a PO box, you might want to use the street address of your post office, and call your box number an apartment number. This will not work for UPS and other delivery companies that will not deliver to PO boxes; for them, you may need to use the address of a trusted friend or neighbor.

The regulations regarding US Post Office Boxes and PMBs are changing rapidly. A federal regulation is going into effect that would require users of either public or private mail boxes to reveal their true address.

Choose a post office box location that has long hours, so you can pick up your mail at many different times. Also take into account how visible you will be when getting your mail, if someone is trying to watch for you there. Is there just one place to park? Just one door to go in and out?

Have different friends pick up your mail whenever possible, to make it harder for the stalker to spot you coming and going from the box location.

If you want the advantages of both a US Post Office box and a PMB, there's no reason why you cannot have both. You might even be able to set them up so that each points to the other as your "home" address, so that your actual residential address appears with neither one.

You might want to get several post office boxes in different locations, so that you will have several addresses to use, and so that your stalker might be steered to one you seldom go to.

• Mail drops

If you can go to some expense and trouble to set up a virtually impenetrable barrier between your mail and your home, use a mail drop, which is a company that will allow you to send and receive mail using their address. They will forward your mail to a private mail box. You can find these in the Yellow Pages under headings such as mail forwarding services or mailing services.

• Credit agencies

Credit agencies maintain lists of previous addresses, so simply sending them a change of address to a PO box may not be enough—ask them to remove all your prior addresses from your record. The three major credit bureaus are CBI-Equifax, Experian (formerly TRW), and Trans Union.

• Return address

Do not use your return address on the outside of envelopes or packages. You can put your PO box on a slip of paper inside, if you like. Be sure to have enough postage on the item, and the correct address, so that the post office will not need to return it to you.

If the post office insists on a return address, use someone else's—your lawyer, your work, or a friend—or just make up a return address. This is especially important if you do not have a private mailbox.

• **Don't use your name**

To reduce the chances of someone finding out more about you than they need to know, consider using a fake name for informal, unofficial purposes when it is going to be associated with your address, whether it is a private mailbox or not. One stalking victim I know has her magazine subscriptions addressed to "Occupant" at her post office box.

• **Friends and family**

Tell your friends and family not to write your true residential address in address books, Rolodexes, or computer files where it might be stolen.

❖ *A stalker's favorite toy—your phone number*

Most stalkers, sooner or later, use the telephone to get to their targets. If you can keep your stalker from finding out your phone number, you have saved yourself from tremendous annoyance.

If you are someone who is at risk to become the target of a celebrity stalker (a doctor, prominent business person, on-air media personality, and so on), precautions taken in advance will pay big dividends, since you never know when a twisted "fan" may suddenly become a fanatic.

Here are some things you can do to protect your phone number.

Protect Your Phone Number
Get a phone number that is hard to find
Use your phone company services
Give out another number
Use toll free numbers with care; they are not secure
Protect your phone bills
Treat pagers like phones
Friends and family must protect your phone number, too

• **Get a phone number that is hard to find**

Get a phone number that is unlisted AND unpublished, but don't count on it being a complete safeguard. Unpublished means it will not appear in the phone book, but will be available if someone calls information; unlisted means it will not be available even to someone who calls information. There are easy ways for people to find out numbers.

Put your phone in a different name, as if you had a roommate. Make it a name like "Mary Smith," "Maria Hernandez," or whatever will blend in with many other people by the same name in the phone book; this is particularly important if you cannot afford to pay for an unlisted, unpublished number. Use this alias whenever you can for bills and services such as electric, gas, cable, and the Internet.

Ask the phone company to keep your address out of the white pages, out of listings on the Internet, and out of the reverse directory (which lets someone who has an address look up the phone number that goes with it).

This one is particularly good if you are moving and do not want the stalker to get your new number. When you order your new telephone service, tell the phone company that you have never had a telephone before. You will have to pay a hefty deposit for about a year, but nobody, not even a telephone company employee who has been bribed to come up with the information, can find your new phone number just by knowing your old one.

• **Phone company services**

Talk to your local phone company. Ask for the person who is in charge of handling harassing calls, and be sure you are not talking to a salesperson who just wants to sell you expensive features. Find out what your phone company can and cannot do for you, and what conditions have to be met for them to take certain actions, such as tracing calls. Then select the services that seem best for your situation.

Not all of these services are available everywhere, and they may go by different names, but some of them are:

- Password protection. This protects your account, so that simply having your phone number is not enough to get information about your account.
- Caller ID. This allows you to see the phone number of most people who call you. Ask about getting a system that will record 10 or more phone calls, not just the last one, so you can see if he called while you were out.
- Enhanced Caller ID. This allows you to see the name as well as the phone number of most people who call you.

- Complete Blocking phone service. This means that people you call cannot see your phone number, even if they have Caller ID. You can selectively unblock on a call-by-call basis, whenever you want to call someone who you know has Caller ID. In some places, Complete Blocking is called Line Blocking.
- Call Trace (described below).
- Call Block. This allows you to completely prevent calls from phone numbers that you specify; calls from those numbers will not even ring.

If your phone company has the Call Trace feature, here is how you can use it:

1. When your stalker calls, hang up on him.
2. Immediately dial the Call Trace code, usually *57, or 1157 on a rotary; this puts his phone number in a temporary file at the phone company
3. Immediately call the phone company to let them know you have used that service, so they will document it.
4. Then call your local police and tell them about the trace. You won't be given the caller's number, but the police will.
5. Remember to document in your stalking log that you received a call, and used Call Trace.

Even if the police do not seem very interested in these reports, keep using Call Trace. It helps to build a solid case against your stalker for use in court.

• **Give out another number**

If you are asked for a phone number in a situation where you don't want to give yours out and when you don't expect that they will ever use it, for example, when cashing a check or registering with a company on the Internet, you might want to consider taking any of the following actions:

- Give the phone number of your lawyer's office
- Make up a phone number
- Write down a nearby area code not your own with the information number 555-1212
- Write down 800-555-1212, which is the information number for 800 phone numbers

Never, ever put your home phone number on a check, credit application, or other such transaction. Give your work phone number, without commenting about it.

When you give out your work phone number, make it the main number, do not include your own extension.

• **Toll free numbers are not secure**

Call 800, 900, and other toll-free phone numbers ONLY from pay phones. Despite Complete Call Blocking, the person or company that pays for the toll-free call will be able to get your phone number when you call.

• **Protect your phone bills**

Your phone bills, and some other communications from your phone company, will have your (listed or unlisted) phone number on them. Shred those documents, or keep them in a very safe place. One stalker got his victim's unlisted phone number by simply stealing her phone bill from her mailbox. Have your bills sent to your private mail box!

• **Pagers**

It is also possible to get the name and address of a person who owns a pager, if that pager number is known, so treat pager numbers with the same caution as phone numbers.

• **Friends and family**

Have your friends and family who call you long distance call only from pay phones. Otherwise, a really determined stalker could hire a private investigator to get a list of the long-distance calls made on your mother's telephone for the past 3 months, and use that list to find your phone number.

Tell your friends and family not to write your phone number in address books, Rolodexes, or computer files where it might be stolen.

If you have other household members with their own telephone lines, you might want to make them unlisted and protect them as carefully as you do your own phone.

❖ *The key to your identity—your Social Security Number*

The Social Security Number, or SSN, was never supposed to be a universal ID number, but it is rapidly becoming one. With your SSN, a stalker may be able to get information about you from your employer, from credit card companies and banks, and from government agencies such as welfare departments.

In any database that your stalker has access to (or can pay someone to access), the most likely key to your record is your SSN. Using it, he can find out far more about you than you want him to know.

"The very first piece of advice I'd give [to targets] is to zealously safeguard their Social Security number," said Leigh Heron, an experienced private investigator (quoted in Snow's book). "Never give out your SSN unless you are totally convinced the person requesting it has a legitimate and definite need for it. Also, don't allow its use on any document open to public viewing."

Protect Your Social Security Number
Give out a fake SSN sometimes
Get another ID number
Don't use your SSN except for tax purposes
Don't write your SSN down

• Give out a fake SSN

Leigh Heron has more advice for dealing with someone who wants your SSN, but doesn't legally require it: "If, however, a company or individual insists on having your Social Security number, even though there is no legal requirement for you to give it, but not giving it will cause problems you'd rather not have, you might consider using the number 078-05-1120. The Social Security Administration used this number in the 1940s and 1950s as a sample number, and it does not belong to anyone. Also available for use, and not belonging to anyone, are the numbers 987-65-4320 through 4329.

Remember, only use one of these numbers with someone who demands but cannot legally require you to give your Social Security number."

• Get another ID number

If your state uses your SSN as an ID number on your driver's license, find out if they will give you another number instead. In some states, all you have to do is ask; in others, you might have to show that you are in danger and in need of privacy. You may you have to show that you have made police reports or have a restraining order against your stalker.

If your school or employer uses SSNs as ID numbers, ask if they will issue you a different number for privacy reasons. Be polite, but very insistent. You may need to work on this issue for quite some time, and to bring others into the fight with you. Many organizations are learning the dangers of using SSNs as IDs, but many still need to be educated.

• Don't use your SSN

Do not use your SSN on checks, credit cards, or anything but legitimate employer, bank, brokerage, or other financial transactions that must be reported for government or tax purposes.

• Don't write your SSN down

Do not carry your social security card or any paper with your SSN on it in your purse or wallet, where it can be stolen.

Memorize your SSN, so that when you need it for a legitimate purpose, you can produce it from memory, instead of having to look it up from a written source.

❖ *Other personal information—safeguard it like gold*

Once you start to become really conscious of all the instances where people try to demand information about you, you will be amazed at how much potentially dangerous information people voluntarily give out to people they assume (but don't know) to be trustworthy.

Practice saying "I don't give out that information," and learn to use that phrase constantly. When faced with a petty "information Nazi" who tries to insist, insist on speaking to his or her supervisor. Be polite, but firm.

You have a lot to protect…

Information to Protect
Your name
Other family members
Birthdate, mother's maiden name
Passwords or "coded" accounts
Government information
Real estate
Voting records
Pollsters, shopper's cards
Credit cards

• Your name

Whenever possible, use your initial or initials instead of your first name. For example, have your credit cards issued with just your initial, not your whole first name, and use your PO Box as the billing address. This makes it harder for someone to track information about you, particularly if you use fake initials frequently.

If you have a nickname, use it frequently. It may help to keep someone who is looking for you under one name from noticing that you have another.

If you are in the public eye, consider using a professional name that is quite different from your true name. This will make it much harder for a celebrity stalker to find out about you.

• Other family members

Protect the personal information (particularly address, phones, and SSNs) of your spouse, your children, and all other family members as zealously as you do your own.

Warn all your friends, relatives, neighbors, co-workers, landlords, and so on to destroy your personal information, or to protect it, and not to give it out on ANY pretext no matter how convincing.

Tell them not to leave this kind of information in obvious places like address books and wallets, where the stalker could steal it. Stalkers frequently break into the homes of friends and family to get information about their targets.

• Birthdate, mother's maiden name

Keep your date of birth and mother's maiden name private, too. Don't ever use them for bank or computer passwords. If you have already done so, change those passwords at once.

• Passwords or "coded" accounts

Tell telephone and utility companies you want to encode your account with a password. A few weeks after you do this, call up the utility company and ask about a charge on your account. If they do not insist on hearing the password from you, insist on talking with a supervisor. Write letters, if necessary, stressing the importance of your privacy.

Even once the password is in place, check every few months to be sure they still ask for it. You might want to change the password every 6 months.

Many organizations, from medical providers to insurance companies to banks, can invoke policies to make your personal information even more protected than usual. Ask if yours have coded accounts, or methods of making your information available to only those who really need to know.

•   Government information

Find out if your state has a provision in the law that allows stalking victims to have personal information that is usually in the public record, such as car registrations, withheld from public view.

If you have ANY court records at all—misdemeanors, domestic, civil, or criminal—talk to a lawyer about how to get the records sealed, so that the stalker can't find out your address, SSN, or other personal information from those files, which are public documents in most states.

•   Real estate

If you own a condo, a house, or business real estate, it might be prudent to transfer the title to someone you trust.

Talk to a lawyer about setting up a trust and having the trust own all of your property, except your car. Be sure to discuss with the lawyer how easy or hard it will be to hide the identities of the trustees, as well as the beneficiary.

•   Voting records

If you move from one location to another, don't have your voting registration transferred to your new location. If you do not vote for a couple of elections and then register anew, it may break a chain of information that otherwise could be used to follow you.

Or, just don't register to vote. Some people decide that privacy and safety is more important than casting a ballot. If you want to participate in electing public officials, you can volunteer to work on someone's campaign.

• Pollsters, shopper's cards

Never give personal information to pollsters.

Never fill out warrantee cards, sweepstakes forms, or questionnaires of any kind.

Don't use shopper's cards that require you to give out a lot of personal information.

If someone phones you or comes to your door asking for information, refuse to give it to them. If they appear to be a company or government person, insist on calling their office to determine whether they are legitimate. Be sure to look up the phone number yourself, don't just call the phone number they give you.

Do not respond to offers for free coupons or chances to win things.

Do not participate in consumer questionnaires, opinion polls, or any other kinds of surveys, whether written or via telephone or the Internet.

Do not complete shopper's cards.

If you really, really, want to fill out a warrantee card, be sure to use your PO Box address, and fill in only the minimum information needed to establish the warrantee; leave blank all the personal information that the company wants to collect for marketing purposes.

• Credit cards

It may seem impossible, but you can get by in today's world using cash and checks. Credit card records are not always as private as they should be; avoid using them whenever you can.

Interlude 1: What would you do?

In these between-chapter interludes, we'll look at various situations that could happen to you, or a friend of yours, and then look at some ways of dealing with them. All of the interludes are based on situations that have actually happened to real people.

A new employee joins your workgroup. In a few days, she suggests the two of you have lunch, just to be friendly and to get to know one another a bit more. You agree, and the two of you eat together in the company cafeteria.

The next week, she suggests lunch again, and again you eat with her. She seems a bit lost and lonely, and asks your advice about how to handle several situations that have come up at work. Flattered that she values your opinion, you discuss the issues with her and offer advice.

A few days later, she is bubbling with thanks for your good advice, and suggests lunch again. You are particularly busy that day, and turn down her offer, though you are glad to have helped her adjust to her new job.

Over the next month, she often presses you to lunch together. When you decline, she immediately says, "How about tomorrow?" When you accept, she fills the conversation with her work problems, which you are starting to tire of helping her solve.

As you decline more and more often, saying that you are too busy, she steps up her attempts to meet with you at other times, suggesting after work get-togethers, dropping notes on your desk, and sending email, pleading for your help.

Her demands are making you more and more uncomfortable. She is pushing for you to become a friend or at least a mentor, and you can't see yourself in that role.

What would you do?

Her actions, though persistent and annoying, don't meet the criteria for stalking. Nonetheless, her actions don't feel quite right.

Her refusal to recognize subtle social cues that you aren't interested in her company could simply be the result of an immature or slightly off center personality.

Some more explicit communication and boundary setting is definitely called for here, such as telling her that you the two of you can lunch together once a month, but not more. Suggest several other people in the office who might be suitable mentors to help her with her job. You might also say that you don't want to meet her outside of work, because you don't mix business relationships with personal ones.

Then, stick to your position, even if it means ignoring her email and requests for help.

Be prepared for her to push back for a while. If she then drops her efforts to monopolize your time, you can consider the problem solved. If instead she continues to ignore your boundary-setting, then stronger steps, may be needed. You might want to start keeping her email and written notes, just to have a record in case the situation escalates.

4 Home—Your Refuge or Your Stalker's Playground?

Keeping personal information safe is an important way to foil stalkers, but there are many aspects of physical safety that are equally important.

There are documented examples of stalkers who gave up on their original intended targets, because they found them "too inaccessible," and so they turned to other victims who could be more easily approached.

In most cases, the number one thing the stalker wants is contact with you. Seeing you in public or through a window at home, hearing your voice on the telephone, knowing you got the "gifts" he sent you—these are his rewards. By denying him these things, you take control of the situation, and he may become discouraged enough to leave you alone.

In a smaller number of cases, the stalker may want to physically harm you. In this situation, you can again take control and deny him that possibility, by making yourself a "hard target," (that is, an extremely difficult target).

The biggest benefit to making yourself a hard target is that every step you take to increase your safety will, after it becomes a normal part of your daily life, make you feel less afraid.

Take extra precautions to make sure that your home is as safe as possible from break-ins and lurkers. There are many books on this subject—your public library can help you find them. The safety measures intended for protection against burglars work just fine against stalkers, too. There are a huge number of things you can do, from inexpensive and unobtrusive to expensive and obvious.

There are three goals to protecting your home. One is to make it difficult for the stalker to know where you live. The second is to make it very difficult for the stalker to break in, whether you are at home or not. The third is to be absolutely certain that if he does break in while you are at home, you will have plenty of warning, and plenty of pre-planned, rehearsed actions you can take to ensure your safety.

When you have achieved those three goals, you can once again relax in your home, instead of being hypervigilant and living in fear.

Safety in and around Your Home
If you rent...
Get the landlord's help
Install safety equipment
Put the rental agreement in another name
Do not put names on the door or mailbox
Park safely
If you live in a house or condo...
Increase lighting, reduce shrubbery
Install peepholes
Lock the fusebox
Make your garage as safe as your house

Make your house number visible
Changing your home environment...
Use interior lights wisely
Install good door locks
Secure the windows
Consider a dog
Consider a home security system
Keep emergency equipment ready
Have multiple ways out
Create a "safe room"
Prepare a mobile emergency kit
Enlist the help of others
Teach your children safety
Coming and going from home...
Prepare your home before you leave it
Use caution when you return; search carefully
Keep doors and windows locked

❖ *If you rent*

• Get the landlord's help

See if you can enlist your landlord's or building manager's help in installing better locks or additional security devices.

If you are not getting the cooperation from your landlord that you need, check with the police, a lawyer, or a tenant's organization to find out what property owners must do, legally, regarding safety issues.

• Safety equipment

Many door and window locks and other kinds of security equipment do not require permanent installation, so you can use them in rental property. Check out your local Home Depot or other hardware store for a lot of safety options.

• Rental agreement

Have the rental agreement in another person's name—a fictional roommate, perhaps, or a family member.

• No names

Do not put your name on your apartment door.

If you are getting all your mail at a post office box or private mail box, don't put your name on your apartment mailbox; use a fake name.

• Parking

If you park in a parking garage or lot, try not to park in the same area all the time. If you have an assigned parking place, make arrangements to occasionally exchange places with another tenant, or to park wherever visitors would park.

Particularly if you have to park in an assigned parking spot in a condo or apartment lot, get in the habit of cruising the entire area to look for suspicious people before pulling into your spot.

See more car-related suggestions in Chapter 6.

❖ *If you live in a house or condo*

• Increase lighting, reduce shrubbery

Along with cars, houses are often a target of a stalker's vandalism. Be sure yours has outdoor lighting, and keep bushes or other "hiding places" as uninviting as possible.

Be sure your front entrance is visible to your neighbors, so they can easily see any suspicious activity going on. If you have a hedge or fence around your property, keep it under 4 feet high, so it cannot easily hide an intruder.

If you want shrubbery in a place that might not enhance security, consider thick, thorny plants that will discourage anyone from hiding in it, or pushing through.

Keep the outside of your home well lit at night. You can get lights that automatically turn on at dusk. Either let the lights stay on all night, or install a motion detector that will turn them on when movement is detected. Dogs and other animals should not set them off, if they are properly adjusted. To keep them from being removed, install them high.

• Peepholes

Install peepholes on your front and back doors. Get the new "panoramic" kind with the widest view angle. If you have children, install the peephole low enough for the children to use, or provide them something secure to stand on so they can use the peephole.

• Electrical security

Is your fusebox accessible? You might want to lock it shut with an inexpensive padlock.

• Garages

Garages can be very dangerous places. Electric garage door openers are worth the money; you don't have to get out of your locked car until you are safely in a locked garage!

Give the lights, shrubs, and other aspects of security where you park the same care you give your house.

• Make your house number visible

Be sure your street number is easily visible from the street, day and night. This will help to ensure that someone calling the police to report trouble can give them the right address, and it will also help the police to find your house quickly. (If you stalker shows up in front of your house, he already knows the address, so making the number visible here is not endangering you.)

❖ *Make your home "unfriendly" to intruders and watchers*

• Interior lights

To make it harder for your stalker to see your movements inside the house at night, position interior lamps so that they are near the windows. This will minimize the shadows you make on curtains or blinds as you walk around inside.

To help keep your stalker out when you are not at home, consider having several lights on timers, to go on and off in patterns that would indicate more than one person is living there. Change the times and patterns frequently, to make it difficult for him to establish what your routines are. Consider leaving a light on in the bathroom all night sometimes—that is very likely to convince a late night visitor that you are awake, and hence that this is not a good time to break in.

• Door locks

If your stalker, or anyone close to him, has ever had a key to your home, change the locks.

Get a good dead bolt lock for each exterior door.

Good door locks are essential. This may require a bit of work, as the best lock in the world is useless if the door is so thin that a booted foot can kick right through it. The screws on the side opposite the lock must be at least 2 inches long to make the door secure.

An excellent defense against a door being kicked in is a metal bar that goes from the doorknob to the floor at an angle. There are many of these "wedge" bars on the market; the best ones allow you to put them in place or remove them, one-handed, in just a second. This ease of use makes it more likely that you will use the bar frequently, and also makes it safer if you have to leave in a hurry because of a fire.

Don't hide an emergency key outside.

Can you live without a mail slot? If so, fasten yours permanently closed.

Put a lock on the inside of your bedroom door, and maybe other bedrooms or interior rooms as well. It should NOT fasten with a key, as you want to be able to get out quickly in case of fire, but it will be a very important barrier against anyone who is trying to get to you.

•   Windows

Secure windows with security pins or bars and put a dowel in the track of all sliding glass doors. Better yet, get a locking bar. Get the kind of window locks that let you open the windows a few inches to get fresh air.

•   Dogs

Should you buy a dog? A dog can be an excellent early warning system, but don't count on one, not even one of the "aggressive" or "protective" breeds, to protect you unless both you and the dog get some very specialized training, which can be expensive. Training must also be practiced regularly or your dog will forget what to do.

Many communities require dogs to be licensed, and you may not want to reveal your address that way. Dogs have to be walked several times a day; will that fit with the part of your security plan that says your activities should be unpredictable?

Also, owning a dog is a very big commitment, one that you should not undertake unless you understand and accept the responsibilities. The long term costs of food and vet bills can be surprisingly high, so be sure you can afford the dog before you get it.

A dog can be an excellent addition to a security plan, but it should never be considered a substitute for good home security, personal awareness, or defensive tools.

• Security Systems

Consider getting a home security system. There are many kinds, from inexpensive motion detectors you can install yourself to incredibly expensive ones that involve Central Station monitoring. Don't buy more than you need or can afford.

Probably the most important feature is to be sure that when you are at home at night, you will be wakened by any kind of intrusion. Your second priority, probably, is protecting the property when you are not at home.

It may be expensive, but you might want to consider a security camera placed in your home or outside to catch the stalker leaving "gifts," vandalizing property, or invading your home. These cameras are very small and unobtrusive, and can be mounted easily.

• Emergency equipment

Keep several flashlights with working batteries in different locations around your home, so you will not be left in the dark if he manages to cut your power.

If you have a gun at home, be sure it is inaccessible to children; not just put where you think they won't find it, but locked up. See Chapter 10 for some suggestions on how to make a defensive gun instantly accessible to you but not to unauthorized users. All responsible adults in the household should have training in the use of the firearm.

Have one or more fire extinguishers in your house, and one in your car or garage.

• Have ways out

Get an emergency escape ladder; you can buy one in the same department as fire extinguishers. Consider getting them for your kids' rooms, too.

In each room, try to envision two different routes of escape, even if they involve things like throwing a chair through a window to create an exit.

Decide how you would get out of your home in several different kinds of emergencies, and practice those routes from time to time.

• Create a "safe room"

Designate one room of your home as the "safe room." This will usually be your bedroom, but might be a child's room. It is the place you and your family will go to immediately if there is danger in the house.

The safe room should have a deadbolt lock that you can close from the inside. Have a cellphone in that room, so that you can call the police even if the stalker has cut the telephone wires to your home. Also have a set of house keys there, so that you can throw them out the window to the police who will be responding to your call. Finally, keep in the safe room whatever weapons you are comfortable using and are trained with.

If you hear a "bump in the night," or even a noise at noon, don't investigate it! Get into your safe room, lock the door, take cover with your weapons at the ready, and phone the police.

• Emergency kit

You might want to put together an "emergency kit" to keep on hand, in case you have to leave in a big hurry. The kit might contain:

- clothes and toiletries for several days
- medications and medical records
- insurance papers
- some money or a credit card or ATM card
- some identification
- a copy of any restraining order you have
- the names, addresses, and phone numbers of several places you could go at any time of the day or night, such as women's shelters or friends houses
- copies of keys for car, home, and work
- originals or photocopies of important ID cards such as driver's license, work ID, voter registration card, welfare ID, green card, your birth certificate, your children's birth certificates, Social Security Card, health insurance card, driver's license, work permits, or passport.

If this sounds like too much to risk keeping in your home or car where your stalker could find it, let a trusted friend or relative keep your emergency kit for you, or keep some of this material in a safe deposit box in a bank.

• Enlist the help of others

Does your neighborhood have a Neighborhood Watch organization? If so, use it. If not, you might want to start one. Talk to your local police to find out how.

Assuming you can trust them, tell your landlord, your close friends, and your neighbors about the stalker. Show them a picture if you have one. Describe his car if you know what it is like. Be sure to warn them not to give out personal information about you to ANYONE, no matter how reasonable or urgent, the request is.

•   If you have children

Teach your children how to call the police and the fire department.

Establish a code word or phrase with your children, and with close friends and family, that means "I'm in trouble! Call for help!"

If your children are old enough, tell them just enough about your situation so that they will understand why you are so careful with personal information, why they must be, too. You don't want to frighten them about your safety or their own, but they deserve some sort of explanation when they observe their parent "lying" about things like their phone number and address.

❖ *Coming and going from home*

•   Before you leave home

When you go out, especially in the evening, put lights, radio, and TV on timers.

If you want to make it difficult for someone to hide in your home waiting for you to return, make the best hiding places inhospitable. Leave closet doors open, put a light in the back of the closets that you can turn on from a safe distance, or have those lights on a timer.

Do not use dust ruffles or bedspreads that fall to the floor and hide under-bed areas. If you must use them anyway, get under-bed storage boxes to fill up the area under your bed, so there isn't room for someone to hide there.

• When you return home

When you come home, have your key in your hand as you approach the door, so you don't have to stand around searching for it.

You might want to establish ways of communicating with your family and neighbors. For example, one light tap on the car horn could just mean "I'm home, please watch while I'm walking to the door," while two beeps could mean "I see the stalker—call the police!"

Don't touch any suspicious-looking package, especially one with no return address, one with a return address you do not recognize, or one that may have been "hand delivered" to your home. A Massachusetts woman was killed by a pipe bomb in a package that was probably left by her stalker. The US Post Office has guidelines for recognizing package bombs; become familiar with them.

If you have a wearable alarm that you remove when you go out, put it on the moment you come through the door, before you even take your coat off.

If you return home and there are obvious signs that someone has been inside, remember that he may still be there. Don't go in! Go to another location and call the police.

If there are no obvious signs of an intruder, you may want to search your home whenever you return. To do this as safely as possible, you should have either your best weapon, or a cellphone ready to speed dial 911, in one hand; use your other hand to open doors. Use all your senses when searching, go very slowly, and pay attention to anything that seems wrong or out of place. If you see or hear something suspicious, don't get close to it. Leave the area and phone the police.

• While you are at home

Keep all of your doors locked whenever you are home. Windows too, if you can.

Close the curtains or shades in windows that a loiterer can see from outside.

When a repair person comes to your home, even if you were expecting him or her, ask for identification.

5 The One Place You Have To Be—At Work

For most people, changing jobs to get away from a stalker is not an option (though if you are considering it, be sure to plan all of the precautions that you would take if you were moving your residence).

One of the most famous instances of workplace stalking started in 1984, when Laura Black was a 22-year-old engineer at a company called ESL in California. Richard Fairly, another engineer at the same company, tried to date her. She declined. He persisted. And persisted. And persisted.

He sent letters (over 200 in 4 years) and gifts. He broke into the company's personnel records to get information about her. He followed her to and from work, and to and from leisure activities. Black moved 3 times trying to escape him, but each time he found her again.

In 1986, ESL fired Farley for his harassment of Black. He became even more threatening.

On February 16, 1988, Farley brought a hundred pounds of guns and ammunition to ESL. He murdered 7 ESL employees, and injured 4 others (including Black). He kept police at bay for more than 5 hours, but was eventually talked into surrendering. He was tried, and sentenced to death in California.

Laura's story was made into a TV movie, "The Stalking of Laura Black."

Whether your stalker first encountered you at work or not, work is the one place where he can be quite sure that you will be, most of the time, so it is natural for him to look for you there. Fortunately, there is a lot you can do to make it hard for him!

Be Safe at Work
Change your work environment, not your job:
Enlist the co-workers you can trust
Consider a company restraining order
Have your employer help
Remove personal information from view
Plan ahead for emergencies
Things to do every day:
Be hard to find
Be extra alert coming and going

❖ Change your work environment, not your job

• Enlist the co-workers you can trust

Tell your boss, your personnel department, and your company's security department about the stalker, and your co-workers if you think they are trustworthy. Show them a picture if you have one. Describe his car if you know what it is like. Warn them not to give out personal information about you to anyone, no matter how reasonable or urgent, the request seems to be.

If you talk frequently with a co-worker, such as a dispatcher, on the phone or radio, you might want to use an alias, so the stalker will not hear your name if he manages to overhear the conversations.

• Company restraining orders

In some states, employers can get restraining orders to keep a stalker at bay. This means that your employer can take steps to enforce the order, and can appear in court instead of you to face the stalker. It may also make it easier for the restraining order to be enforced.

For example:

- Continental Airlines filed suit against the ex-wife of a Continental pilot, because she had baked him a loaf of rye bread with marijuana in it, trying to get him fired by failing a drug test.
- Polaroid obtained a restraining order to help protect an employee who was being stalked. Polaroid will also tap the phone of any employee being stalked, and will even post security guards at their home.
- I have been told by people in the security organization at Fidelity Investments and at GTE Internetworking that those companies would obtain restraining orders to help protect an employee who was being stalked.

Find out if this is possible in your state, and find out if your company is willing to help you in this way.

• Other things your employer might do

Try to get some flexibility in the times you can arrive at work and leave. so you are not coming and going predictable.

Have someone else record your phone answering message, or use the company-provided generic one, so that the stalker will not get the "reward" of hearing your voice if he calls you at work.

If the stalker knows the location of your office or work area, try to get it moved. One stalker drove his car through an exterior wall, into the office that his victim had occupied until a few days earlier, when she moved upstairs to make it harder for him to find her.

• Remove personal information

Remove personal information, including your name, from as many places as possible. If you are lucky enough to have a named parking place, take your name off it, or give it to someone else so you don't park in the same place every day. Take the nameplate off your locker or door, the name sign off your desk; use a fake name if necessary.

Keep your business cards in a drawer instead of in a holder on your desk.

Don't have any photos of your family at work.

Don't have any personal information about you or your family visible or where someone searching your work area would find it easily.

If you use a computer at work, check the tips in the section on Safety with Computers.

• Plan ahead

Consider how you would get out of your work area in an emergency. Try to have at least two possible exits in mind from all the places you are during your workday.

If you can, set up your phone to speed dial an emergency number (the police, or your company security) with the minimum number of button pushes. Test your memory occasionally by going through the motions, without actually pushing the buttons. Remember to practice dialing a "9" if that is required to get an outside line.

• Working at home

If you work out of your home, do not use your residential address on stationery, business cards, envelopes, and so on. Use your post office box or private mail box instead.

❖ *Things to do every day*

• Be hard to find

If possible, have your phone calls, mail, packages, and visitors screened by someone else.

Do not let your name be used on whiteboards, bulletin boards, maps, wall displays, or other places where your stalker might be able to glean information about you.

Vary your schedule as much as possible. Don't eat lunch at the same time or in the same place every day. Vary your break times if possible.

Try not to be the only person in the bathroom.

• Coming and going

Ask company security personnel or co-workers to walk with you to your car.

Park in different places in the parking lot.

Especially if you use public transportation, try to come and go at slightly different times, so he cannot follow you easily.

Occasionally come to work in one set of clothes, and change into another before you leave.

Have your best weapon (phone, Persuader, pepper spray, etc.) in your hand in your coat pocket when you come and go from work.

Stay in a state of relaxed awareness (Chapter 1) when you are coming and going from work.

Interlude 2: What would you do?

You accept a date with a guy you don't know very well. You met him at a party at a friend's house, and he seems just like a regular guy, so you gave him your phone number when he asked.

A few nights later, he calls and suggests dinner, and then a movie that you really want to see. Pleased, you accept. Being the cautious type, you arrange to meet him at the restaurant, so you don't have to tell him where you live.

Over dinner, he is funny and charming. The two of you find several interests in common, and have a pleasant meal. The movie is fun, too, and you feel relaxed enough to let him deliver you to your door, and you invite him up for coffee.

Once in your apartment, he changes subtly, not pushing for any physical closeness, but acting more like someone in his own home than a guest in someone else's. He ignores your hints that it is getting very late, and you finally have to ask him to leave. With obvious reluctance, he does. "He's a bit of a boor," you think.

In the next few weeks, he calls several times to ask you out, but by then you have met someone else you are more interested in, and you turn him down.

He sends you flowers, and a teddy bear holding a sign that says "You are wonderful!" You thank him, but you also tell him explicitly that you do not want to go out with him again.

Over the next 5 or 6 months, he calls you every few weeks, asking you out, and sends 4 more presents. You refuse his requests (or simply let the answering machine take them), and you stop acknowledging his presents. His persistence is flattering, but it is also starting to annoy you.

Late one night, he calls you, waking you up from a sound sleep. He begs you to let him come over, because he needs to talk to you. You refuse to see him, and very firmly get off the phone and go back to sleep. A half hour later, your are awakened from sleep again, this time by the doorbell ringing. Sure it is him, you ignore it. He stops leaning on the doorbell, and eventually you manage to go to sleep again. This time, nothing about the situation felt flattering. You feel uneasy that he came to your home unbidden, and you are angry that he ruined your night's rest.

In the morning, as you go to your car, a neighbor stops you to say that he noticed a car driving around and around and around your building for many hours last night. He describes the car, and it sounds just like your would-be suitor's car. Your unease turns to real concern, as you look around for further signs of him, thinking "I wish he didn't know where I live! What am I going to do now?"

What would you do?

His behavior is definitely over the line of acceptable, but if someone asked you if you were being stalked, you would probably say, "Of course not. He is boorish, persistent, and even childish, but he's not a stalker."

He has certainly exhibited a pattern of unwanted behavior over a period of many months. You have been consistent in your message to him that the relationship between you, if there ever was one, has no future, and he has not listened to that message.

Let's not quibble about whether this is stalking or not. The answer might, in fact, depend on the law in your area. But whether it is stalking or not, his escalated attempts to reach you are causing real concern.

At this point, you might start telling your friends, and the neighbor who was interested enough in your welfare to tell you about the suspicious vehicle, what has been going on. Let them start being additional eyes and ears, to spot this guy if he comes around again. Ask your neighbor to call the police if that car starts circling your building again.

This would also be a good time to review your overall safety situation at home (and at work, if he knows where you work), to think about changing your phone number to an unlisted one, and to start noticing whether he might be following you when you leave one or the other. If you haven't been keeping a log of his contacts and actions, this is a great time to start one, beginning with as detailed a history as you can remember.

6 Going For A Ride—Your Car

Do you feel safe in your car, or vulnerable? Probably both, depending on what is going on around you.

Vulnerability often comes from the feeling that the stalker might easily force you off the road, or follow you home.

One of the people who AWARE trained was followed by her ex-husband, who tried to force her off the road. Another woman who contacted AWARE for assistance felt she was frequently followed when she was driving. Both women were unharmed, but their situations show that stalking victims need to be especially alert and careful in cars.

Safety can come from the knowledge that you are in a multi-ton shelter that can double very nicely as a mobile weapon, if necessary, to save your life.

Here are some ways you can increase your safety, and decrease your vulnerability.

Be Safe in your Car
In and around your vehicle:
Have everything you might need
Keep your car anonymous
Use different cars
Plan before you drive
Driving safely:
Approach your car alertly
Be alert when you drive
Follow safety habits as you drive
If you are followed, go to a crowded place
Park safely
Practice defensive driving
Be careful with kids in cars
In an emergency, drive away. If you can't, stay in the car and use the horn!

❖ *In and around your vehicle*

• Have everything you might need

Keep your gas tank full, and your car in good operating condition.

Keep a pen or pencil and a small notebook in your car, so you can write down any suspicious license numbers or vehicle descriptions.

Keep a flashlight with working batteries in your car where you can reach it easily, not in the trunk. It should be powerful enough to illuminate things and people outside the car.

Have a telephone available to you whenever you are in your car, a cell-phone in your purse or pocket is your lifeline.

Stalkers often vandalize cars. Get a gas cap that locks, and is unlockable only from within the car, to make it harder for him to add sugar or other substances to your gas tank.

Be sure you have a spare tire, and the tools and knowledge necessary to change a tire. (But if you have a flat and think it isn't safe to get out of the car, go ahead and drive on the flat. Better a ruined tire than a ruined life.)

Have a blanket ("space blankets" don't take much room), gloves, and some warm clothes in your car.

• Keep your car anonymous

Don't have vanity plates, bumper stickers, or other distinctive markings on your car that make it easier to identify or follow.

If you must keep your automobile registration in the car, don't keep it in an obvious place such as the glove box or above the sun visor.

Do not put your name, your car license number or any other information that would identify your car your key chain.

Do not leave things in your car that you don't want your stalker to see. For example, when you pick up mail, don't leave it visible in the car; you may be encouraging in a break-in.

• **Use different cars**

You might want to go so far as to get a different car, to make it harder for your stalker to find you.

If that is too extreme, or too expensive, borrow a friend's car from time to time, so you aren't always in the same vehicle.

If you rent a car, be sure the rental company does not have your actual address or telephone number. A particularly resourceful stalker got his target's home address by breaking into the rental car office she had used.

• **Plan before you drive**

If you are going to take a trip, or drive to any place that is new to you, plan your route carefully in advance. There are several places on the Internet that will print maps and directions for free; try http://www.expedia.com, http://www.vicinity.com/geocities/driving.html or http://www.mapquest.com/ If you are a AAA member, you can get maps from them at no cost. Have maps and directions with you so you won't have to stop and get out of the car to ask.

❖ *Driving safely*

•   Going to your car

When you approach your car, notice the vehicles around it. If there is a van on the driver's side, you might want to get in from the passenger side.

Always glance under, around, and in your car, especially in the back seat, before you get in it.

When you approach your car, have your keys in your hand (your hand can still be in your purse or pocket) so that you do not have to stand at your car fumbling to find the keys.

Most assaults at cars come from the rear of the car. To avoid this, or to give yourself the maximum amount of time to react, learn to unlock the door and open it with your left hand. This will position you so that you can easily see the back of the car and whatever is beyond it; it also makes it very hard for anyone to push you into the car.

Get in the habit of locking the car doors the moment you get in the car, before you put on your seat belt or start the car.

As soon as you have locked the door, drive away. Don't sit around reading, or checking your packages, or searching through your purse.

If you have kids, don't leave them alone in the car, not even while you return a shopping cart across the parking lot. You don't want your stalker to have the idea of getting at you by getting at your children!

If someone is coming after you as you get into the car, the most important thing to do is lock the door. Then drive away as fast as you safely can, while leaning on the horn!

If you are being attacked at your car, and you don't have enough time to get into the car, drop to the ground and crawl under the car. Yell, kick and bite viciously, and deploy whatever weapons you have.

• When you are driving

Keep the windows up whenever you are in the car. If it is too hot that way, open both the front and rear windows on the same side of the car just a few inches, not enough for someone to reach inside. This will give you air circulation, but not wind.

Keep the doors locked!

Vary your routes and departure times to and from work and the places you shop. In fact, vary the places you shop and use for recreation as much as possible, so the stalker cannot find you by hanging out around your usual grocery store, ATM, movie theater, swim club, mall, etc.

When stopping in traffic, make sure you can see the road between the front of your car and the back of the car in front. This will give you enough space to maneuver around that car, if someone comes up to the car to attack or harass you while you are stopped.

While you are stopped, remember to stay in a state of "relaxed awareness," don't "space out."

Keep your radio at a volume which allows you to hear activity around your car.

• If you are followed

If you think someone might be following you, don't try to speed away from him. That would be dangerous to you and any other drivers and bystanders, and it will only encourage your follower to keep after you. Also, don't slam on the brakes. He won't be intimidated, and you have nothing to gain by causing a crash.

Find a place where you can go around the block or take some other roads to go in a circle, watching whether the vehicle you suspect makes all the same turns. If it does, you know for sure that you are being followed.

If you have a cellphone, this would be a good time to use it to call the police!

Whether you have called the police or not, do not continue to drive to your original destination! Instead, drive to a police station, fire station, hospital, 24 hour store, shopping center, gas station or other busy area where people are guaranteed to be. (At some police stations, there won't be many people around, since most people on shift do not sit around the station.)

When you get to the safe, busy area, don't get out of your car! Stay there, flash your headlights, and blow the horn to attract attention.

Even if you evade your pursuer and make it home unharmed, report the incident to the police. Give as much detail as you can about the car that followed you, and the person or people in it.

• When you park

When you park, always think about what it will be like to come back to the car later, and choose your parking spot accordingly. Park near an attendant, near a light source, or near an exit.

If you possibly can, back into the parking space, so that you will not have to back out when you leave.

Do not use parking services where you have to give your key to someone to park it for you. It is too easy for someone to get to your key if it is inadequately secured. If you must use this type of service, give the attendant just your car key, not your whole keychain.

• Defensive driving

Learn defensive driving techniques from a reputable driving academy, one that teaches police or professional bodyguards. There is more on this in the self-defense chapter.

• Kids in cars

When you return to your car from shopping, get your kids into the car before you put your purchases in. That way, there is less chance that someone will go after them while you are occupied with groceries.

• Handling emergencies

Stay in the car! Use the horn!!!

A moving target is harder to hit, so keep your car moving if at all possible.

If you have a cellphone in your car, remember that if you call for help, the police will not know where you are unless you tell them your exact location.

If you are in a minor traffic accident, remember that your stalker, or a friend of his, may have caused it to force you out of your car. Don't fall for it! In the car is the safest place for you to be, so stay in the car, open the window only an inch to exchange insurance paperwork. Use your cellphone to call police or to call a tow truck.

Do not stop to assist a stranded motorist; he (or she) may be a decoy for your stalker. If you want to help, use your cellphone to call the police to report the location of the stranded car.

If you are in danger from someone who is outside your car, don't get out of your car! Use your car to escape—drive over him if he would kill you otherwise. Drive to where there are other people, and use your car's horn to attract attention.

If you are in danger from someone who is in your car, don't let him take you anywhere—being kidnapped will put you in far more danger than you already are. Refuse to drive. Refuse to give him the keys. Throw the keys far outside the window if necessary. If both of you are in the car, a good technique is to turn sideways with your back against the car door, lift both legs to your chest, and "bicycle kick" the would-be kidnapper repeatedly as hard and fast as you can, preferably hitting him with your heels. If he is driving, cause an accident by gouging his eyes, or yanking the steering wheel so the car crashes into something that will stop it.

7 Public Places—Is There Safety in Numbers?

Public places can often feel safer than private ones, since few stalkers are crazy enough to initiate a violent attack in the presence of witnesses. Some stalkers are that deranged, however. Arthur Jackson stabbed actress Theresa Saldana 10 times in the street in front of her apartment building, very nearly killing her, before a nearby delivery man managed to pull the crazed attacker away.

Even stalkers who refrain from violence may be more than willing to follow or otherwise annoy and frighten their targets in public.

"Public" places can become suddenly and unexpectedly devoid of other people, turning them into dangerous, frightening, solitary places.

Knowing how to maintain relaxed awareness in public places will help you keep your life as normal as possible, while still staying safe.

Be Safe in Public
Have an escape route
Don't be predictable
Keep your defensive tools handy
Be alert when you walk. Keep moving!
If you are approached, respond appropriately
Use caution in busses, subways, trains, and taxis
Ask for assistance

❖ *Be prepared*

• Have an escape route

Wherever you are, always be prepared to escape to safety. In restaurants, stores, and everywhere else, as soon as you go in, notice where the exits are.

Know where "safe places" are in your neighborhood. Which stores are open late, or all night? Where is the police department? The fire department?

• Don't be predictable

Vary your routine. Use different ATMs in different locations, at different days and times. Shop at different stores. Visit different restaurants and bars. Go to different movie theaters.

Find new organizations to be part of, such as a place to worship and a new health club.

• Defensive tools

Depending on your level of training, and what is legal where you live, you might have several defensive tools with you, such as a noise-maker (air horn or electronic "screamer"), a Persuader, pepper spray, or even a firearm. Your best defensive tool is your brain, but having at least two other tools handy is a good idea. You might decide, for example, to put your Persuader in your waistband, and your pepper spray in your coat pocket.

❖ *On foot*

• Walking around

Wherever you walk, keep your head up and your eyes and ears open. Be aware of who is around you at all times.

Do not wear headphones; they make it much harder for you to realize that someone is approaching you.

Wear shoes you can run in, if necessary.

Walk in the center of the sidewalk, not on the edge near traffic, nor on the side near doorways.

Try not to be alone. Shop with a friend!

A moving target is harder to hit. Try to keep moving at all times, especially if you are nervous. If someone asks you for the time, or directions, or any other question, just keep walking as you say firmly "I don't know."

Walk with your hands empty, so you can easily start to fight or reach for a weapon if you need to.

• If you are approached

If you feel threatened by someone who is approaching you, briefly look directly at him so he knows you have seen him, and take evasive action. Go into the street if there isn't much traffic, or head for the nearest populated place.

❖ *Public transportation*

• Busses, subways, and trains

Know the schedules, and have a schedule with you always.

If possible, vary your comings and goings so you don't take the same transportation from the same place at the same time every day.

Try to arrive at the stop shortly before the bus, train, or subway arrives, so you don't have to stand around and wait.

If you do have to wait, try to do it near a guard booth or toll window. If there are no officials around, wait where other people can see you, but not too close to those other people.

Figure out where you would go for assistance if you had to get off a few stops early, or if you stayed on beyond your normal stop.

• **Taxis**

If you take taxis and are at all uncomfortable about the driver, do not get in.

Don't share taxi rides with strangers.

• **Ask for assistance**

On busses, subways or trains, sit as near to the driver as possible.

If you use the transportation system frequently, explain your situation to someone in charge, and find out if there are any special services you might be able to use, such as having a bus driver let you off at a non-standard stop, or letting you sit in the "reserved" seats near the driver.

If you feel uncomfortable or threatened by anyone, don't keep it to yourself. Tell someone in charge, or your fellow passengers if necessary, what is going on.

❖ *Bicycles*

A bicycle is a great method of transportation. You can easily outdistance someone running behind you, and you can zip into places where a car following you can't follow. But you are vulnerable to larger vehicles, and you have no protection around you in the form of lockable doors and closeable windows.

Unlocking a bike from a bike rack and getting underway is inherently a slower, more exposed activity than getting into a car, so you need to be extra aware of who is around before you approach your bike.

Look around the places you frequently bike in, and make advance plans about where you would go if you feel threatened.

If you have defensive tools, be sure to carry them where they will be accessible without dismounting your bike. Pepper spray in your backpack isn't going to do you any good at all.

Many of the same rules apply to bikes as cars: don't let yourself be stopped or distracted; always have a plan; always be aware of who is around you.

8 Cyber Safety—Is It Possible?

Gary S. Dellapenta, 50-year old security guard from North Hollywood, met a woman at church who rebuffed his romantic advances. How did he get back at her? He put ads in her name on American Online, Hotmail, and other Internet sites; the ads described fantasies of being gang-raped.

When people responded, he revealed personal information about her, from the address of her apartment to her physical description, her phone number, and how to bypass her security system.

He became the first person prosecuted under California's cyber-stalking law; the charges included stalking, computer fraud, and solicitation of sexual assault.

Many of the suggestions in this section have to do with preserving your computer privacy before someone seriously invades it, but if you know you have a stalker, or even if someone is just making you feel antsy, you need to be very, very careful.

These suggestions are for computers at home or at work, with or without Internet access.

Be Safe Using Your Computer
Don't show personal information
Protect your passwords
Encrypt sensitive documents
Enlist the help of your ISP
Make your browser anonymous
Use caution sending email
Save and report harassing email; don't answer it!
Be cautious when buying things on-line
Assume your stalker is in your chat rooms
Learn more about privacy

❖ Your computer

• Don't show personal information

If someone glances at your computer when you are gone for a moment, is it obvious that it is yours?

Don't name your computer after yourself, don't have family photos as backgrounds or screensavers, and don't give folders or files names like "Terri's notes" or "Stalking log."

• Passwords

Be sure your passwords are not easy to guess. One way to create a password that is easy to remember but hard to guess is to use the first letter, number, or punctuation in each word in a favorite saying, song, verse, or poem. For example, if you know you will remember the ditty "Three blind mice, see how they run!" then your password can be "3bm,shtr!"

Change your passwords every few months.

Do not use a single password for everything.

• Encrypt sensitive documents

Learn to use encryption software such as PGP (Pretty Good Privacy) when you communicate with friends by email or when you send documents. That way, even if he intercepts your email, he will not have the satisfaction of being able to read it.

You can encrypt files or documents on your computer, as well as email.

❖ *Using the Internet*

• Internet Service Providers

Be sure your Internet Service Provider (ISP) has a policy of never giving out personal information on subscribers unless ordered to do so by a court.

Lexis-Nexis P-Trak service will, for a fee, obtain the address, birthdate, and phone number of individuals. Don't let them give out your information! Whenever you hear of these or other Internet sites that provides information on people, contact the organization and ask that your personal information be removed from their databases.

•   Make your browser anonymous

Did you know that your browser, Netscape or Microsoft Internet Explorer, is probably set to make personal information about you available to others on the Internet? If you have never changed the default settings of your browser, you are vulnerable. To fix this, go into the Preferences section of your browser, find the User (or Personal) information, and remove all personal information, such as your name and email address.

•   Sending email

If you need to browse or send email anonymously, use a service that allows you to do this securely such as www.anonymizer.com

Treat email like a phone call—do not give out any personal information to unknown people who contact you this way.

Consider any email you send to be as visible to the world as a postcard; it is NOT private like a letter. This technology is moving fast. Better safeguards will be available soon, incorporated into browsers and email systems, but don't count on them to do everything you need.

•   Getting threatening or harassing email

If you get harassing email from your stalker, save both hardcopy and electronic versions. Obviously, do not reply or respond in any way.

Contact your ISP for assistance in stopping the harassment. When these problems first started happening, the ISPs were as clueless as anyone else about how to deal with them. Now, most ISPs will, if there is a court order to do so, release information about the owners of accounts who are suspected of harassment. But even without a court order to release information about your stalker, there are things they can do. Contact them, and send copies of the stalker's messages. If they aren't sufficiently responsive, you should consider changing ISPs. (Yes, it is a spot of bother to change your email name and get used to another on-line "home," but it is worth it, particularly if you take more steps to protect your privacy when you switch ISPs than you did when you originally signed up for that first service.)

Contact the FBI. They are knowledgeable about this crime; your local police may or may not be.

• Buying things on-line

If you register with any website, or if you buy things from any on-line service, remember to use your PO box, and use an initial instead of your full first name. If they insist on a phone number and you do not want to give yours, see the chapter on telephones for alternatives.

• Chat rooms

Chat rooms can be fun, but they can be dangerous, too. Stalkers have found many victims that way. The best thing is to avoid using them, but if you must chat, be sure that you don't give out any personal information. Treat every on-line conversation as if your stalker were on the other end. Remember that it is easy for a single person to have multiple identities on the web, so if you mention to one person the name of the town where you live, and later mention to another person the name of the street you live on, you may have just given your stalker the means to find you. Don't divulge any personal information, at all. None!!

• Learn more about privacy

There are some organizations in the resource list in Appendix A about computer privacy, using the Internet safely, and so on. Look at them from time to time to learn the latest suggestions for protecting your privacy, and follow their rules to protect your computer, particularly when you are connected to the Internet.

Interlude 3: What would you do?

When you bought your house, you loved the neighborhood. Your kids could walk to school, and all the neighbors seemed very nice. The 15-year-old boy across the street even agreed to do some yard work for you.

But after you had been there for a few months, you began to think that the neighbor boy was hanging around rather too often, and he seemed to be trying to cultivate a close friendship with your 7-year-old daughter, playing with her and giving her little gifts.

You discouraged the friendship, but the boy persisted, phoning for her several times a day. Of course, you never let her speak to him. He started saying that he wanted your daughter to be his girlfriend when she got older. You talked to his parents, who were quite cooperative and forbade him phone her, or to visit your house or yard. For a month or so, he obeyed. Then the gifts and calls started again. You started driving your daughter to and from school, instead of letting her walk.

Again, you talked to his parents, and again they did their best to crack down. Again, he denied that he has any sexual interest in her, but "just wants to be friends" so she can be his girlfriend someday. A few mornings later, your car, which you parked in your driveway, had two flat tires.

His parents denied that their son could have been responsible for the tires, and continued to try to control him. A few days later, your car's paint was badly scratched, as if a nail had been dragged against it. And the resourceful boy always seemed to be able to find some way to contact your daughter, who was clearly afraid of him, and sometimes cried when the telephone rang, which was 15 or 20 times a day.

You reported the car's vandalism to the police, and told them exactly what had been going on. The boy's parents suddenly became very uncooperative.

What would you do now?

Is this a case of stalking? Just because the boy and the girl are both young doesn't exempt what is going on from that definition. He has clearly been harassing her with unwanted attention repeatedly, over a period of several months. His interest in her, even if it is not sexual, is completely improper, and he does not seem to be able to control his attentions.

The incessant phone calls are just as terrifying to a child as they would be to an adult woman, if not more so. The increased frequency of the phone calls and the escalation of vandalism are also indicators that something very serious is going on, and is getting worse.

This would be a good time to get the police involved, and to find out whether a stalking charge could be brought against the boy. If the police are cooperative, they may be able to impress on him the seriousness of the consequences of his actions. You can do your part by impressing on the boy (and his parents) that you will not hesitate to involve the police if necessary. Perhaps you need a safety review of your house, and a perimeter alarm system so that you cannot have any "surprise" visits from anyone.

Clearly your daughter is being adversely affected by the situation, and needs to know that you will protect her. She is old enough to understand a little of what is going on, so she is old enough to know a little about the actions you are taking, such as getting an unlisted telephone number to make it harder for him to keep calling.

We don't normally think of children as stalkers or stalking victims. When such a situation happens, both families are also involved, and emotions will run high. You probably aren't going to be able to change the boy's behavior much, so don't try. Let his parents and others deal with that issue; you can concentrate on strengthening all of your safety precautions, and getting help by informing other organizations, such as your daughter's school.

9 Using the Telephone—You Thought You Knew How

The telephone is something we all depend on to keep in touch with friends, make plans, get information, and do work. For most people, a ringing telephone, if not a welcome sound, is at worst an annoyance, another one of those telemarketers calling at dinnertime.

But for people who are the targets of stalkers, the telephone can be an instrument of torture! The telephone is one of a stalker's favorite tools; more than a hundred calls a day is not unheard of.

Phone calls don't have to be frequent to be frightening. Even very occasional calls can be terrifying, whether the stalker remains silent, makes demands, threatens, or spouts obscenities. One stalker used to call his target from time to time, just to say that he liked the clothes she was wearing that day. Imagine yourself on the receiving end of calls like that, and you can easily understand why it is important to have a telephone available whenever you need it for an emergency, while minimizing your stalker's ability to annoy or terrify you with that same instrument.

Here are some tips and techniques to reduce your phone-related harassment.

Safety on the Telephone
Don't let him hear your voice
Use an answering system
Fool him with a second line
Prepare for an emergency
Get help from your phone company
Get a cellphone
Friends and family should be cautious
Answer the phone carefully
Be careful with cordless phones
Make calls untraceable
In an emergency, call 911

❖ Don't let him hear your voice

• Use an answering system

Get a telephone answering system, and use it to screen all your calls. Get the mini-cassette type, so you can remove, date, and keep the tapes. If possible, do not get the digital type of answering machine, because, with them, you can only overwrite the messages, not physically remove them and save them for evidence in court.

Have your husband, boyfriend, or a male friend record your answering system message.

Do not use any names, not even first names in your answering message.

What if you cannot afford features like Caller ID or an answering machine? There is still a lot you can do. You can explain your problem to the telephone company and try to get their assistance in tracing the calls. You can keep a journal (log) of when he calls. If he calls back repeatedly, unplug the phone to stop it ringing.

• Fool him with a second line

If you can afford it, leave your current phone number in place, with its cassette answering machine. Get a second phone line, with a new number (unpublished, unlisted, in another name) that you give out only to trusted friends and family. With luck, your stalker will never think to look for a second phone number, and you won't be very bothered by the calls that are recorded on the "stalker line."

• Prepare for an emergency

Post emergency numbers (police, fire, women's shelter, and so on, but not family) near each telephone.

Keep a pen, paper and clock near each phone, so you can note the time and content of any strange calls. Strange calls can be very upsetting, whether you hear the stalker's voice or not. Having a routine to follow when you get one will help you feel in control again.

❖ *Phones and phone companies*

• **Get help from your telephone company**

Telephone company products and features change frequently. Re-contact your phone company about once a year to find out if new services are available that would help you deal with your stalker.

Even without a pre-arranged trace, a phone company might be able to do a "tape search" to identify a call to or from any number in their area. Depending on how long they keep the records, such a search may be good up to 30 or 60 days! To be effective, you must be as precise as possible about the time that the call was made. Phone companies may charge for this service, so find out in advance if they can do it, and how much it costs.

Most phone companies will let you install a phone line in a location other than your residence, and call-forward to a phone in your residence.

• **Get a cellphone**

Cellphone technology is changing rapidly. At the moment, you can get analog or digital, dual or tri-cellphone service. Digital may be the most secure from eavesdropping, but analog probably has the largest service area; dual and tri-phones have both types of signals. You can even get Caller ID on some cellphones. If you are getting a cellphone primarily for emergency calls, you will likely want an analog, dual, or tri one, to minimize the chances of being in a no-service area when your emergency occurs.

If you get a cellphone, protect it and its phone number in the same way as your residential phone. Have the bill sent to your private mailbox, put it in a different name, and be sure there is a password on the account. However, you can give this number out a little more freely than your home phone, because you can turn the phone off whenever you do not want to be called, and because it is harder for the stalker to find your home address from it, even if he finds the cellphone number.

• Cellphones may be available free for emergencies

The Wireless Foundation (of which Verizon Wireless is a member), the National Coalition Against Domestic Violence and Motorola are sponsors of a national program called "Call To Protect." The program helps distribute pre-programmed emergency wireless phones free of charge to victims of domestic violence. These phones can be used for emergency calls only, but they are free. Air time for the emergency calls is donated by local wireless carriers. For more information, see http://www.wirelessfoundation.org, or contact a local organization that helps domestic violence victims.

❖ *Making and receiving calls*

• Friends and family

Many stalkers have pried information out of people close to their target by pretending to be old school friends, delivery people, or any other scam they can think of. Teach your friends and family that when someone they don't know calls them, don't just talk to them—insist on taking their phone number and calling them back.

- ## Answer the telephone carefully

Never answer the phone until the answering machine picks up first, and you are sure the caller is someone you want to talk to.

If you do not have an answering machine, pick up the phone but don't say "Hello." Wait for the caller to speak first. If nobody speaks for about 5 seconds, quietly hang up. Your wanted callers will learn to say something quickly, and you won't reward the stalker with the sound of your voice.

- ## Dialing 911 from a cellphone

In most places, using a cellphone to call 911 will connect you to the state police, or a 911 operator at the state level. Then, after you give them the information about where you are, and what is happening to you, they will relay the call to the local authorities. Always give your location first, then details such as the problem you are having, and your name.

- ## Be wary of cordless phones

Be cautious when using cordless or cellphones; they can be eaves-dropped on much more easily than corded phones. Never discuss any personal information on a cordless or cellphone.

The age of your cordless phone may have a lot to do with how secure from evesdropping it is; newer technology is getting more secure.

You should also be aware that baby monitors can be eavesdropped on, by someone outside your residence with a scanner tuned to the right frequency. Turn the monitor off when not in use, and be careful what you say when it is on.

• Make calls untraceable

Do not use telephone credit cards—it is too easy to trace those records. Keep enough change with you to make the calls you need at pay phones.

To make private calls, use prepaid calling cards. No personal information is required to purchase them.

Borrow a friend's phone, and then pay him or her for the calls, so nothing shows up in your telephone records.

• In an emergency, call 911

Remember, any public pay phone MUST allow you to call for help without having to insert any money first. Dial 911 if your area has that service, or memorize the number of the police department.

All cellphones sold after the year 2002 must be able to automatically give the location of any 911 call. Until then, you must remember to SAY WHERE YOU ARE whenever you dial a 911 or other emergency call from a mobile phone.

10 What Nobody Else Will Tell You About Self-Defense

This section will be quite unlike what has come before. Until now, we have looked at what you can do to prevent contact with your stalker. But what should you do if, despite your best efforts, he breaches your "avoidance" defenses? What should you do if your stalker is one of the 25-30% who become violent, and he becomes violent against you?

You need to learn what you can do to prepare for such a frightening, but survivable situation.

Why should you bother with self-defense, if your stalker hasn't shown any indication of violence? Even if your stalker has never been violent, that could all change in a single hour.

There is no time to take swimming lessons when your boat is sinking—you MUST have learned that life-saving skill in advance. So it is with self-defense.

Much "standard" self-defense information and training is intended to help women protect themselves from rape or street crimes like purse snatching. This is important—learning to fight back physically against a bigger, stronger assailant is incredibly empowering and something everyone should learn—but knowing how to land groin kicks and eye jabs is useless if your stalker conducts his "attacks" by telephone and mail.

Such hands-on defenses are also sub-optimal if your stalker decides to try to kill you; you will need more than a devastating ax kick if he has a gun or a knife.

Schaum and Parrish are big advocates of self-defense. They say, "…taking personal measures toward self-defense…can also go far in helping a victim reclaim strength and reestablish a sense of safety."

Most stalking experts agree that self-defense training is probably a good thing for stalking victims to have, but few resources are available to actually provide an overview of the many kinds of self-defense techniques, and evaluate them with regard to their usefulness in protection from stalkers, so this chapter will go into quite a bit of depth about many different methods and tools.

No book can teach you techniques, however, so this chapter CANNOT show you how to use the different methods discussed here. It will, however, help you select which ones you want to follow up on, and point you to resources for finding qualified instructors in your area. You MUST get formal training!

Avoidance of danger is always your prime objective, and your first responsibility. If you can arrange your life so that your stalker cannot easily find you, you have avoided danger. If you can keep a locked door between you and your stalker, you have avoided danger. If you have time and the opportunity to call highly trained resources, such as the police, to help (and if they can get to you in time), you have avoided danger.

Virtually all the suggestions in this book, up to this point, have had to do with avoiding your stalker, by keeping him away from you and keeping yourself away from your stalker.

So, what should you do if those preventive measures fail, and the stalker is about to physically harm you? In such a terrible situation, the best strategy is to fight back hard and fast, with all your might!

Fight empty-handed or with whatever tools you have in your possession that are appropriate to the situation.

Think you can't fight? You are wrong! All women, as well as men, have a strong, natural urge to survive that brings out an amazingly strong fighting response when attacked. In particular, women who have children generally turn into wolf-women protecting their offspring when anyone seriously threatens their child.

The survival urge, however, must be channeled together with proper training to make an effective self-defense package. Fighting back can be easy, natural, and extremely effective if you have had proper training.

Unfortunately, when it comes to the question of whether stalking victims should arm themselves, some so-called experts give advice that is inconsistent with common sense. "Carrying a weapon is useless if a stalker surprises you," says one well-meaning but uninformed advice-giver. "Having a gun, knife, pepper spray, or electrical shocking device is of no value if the self-defense weapon is not out and ready to use." But that simply doesn't make sense. Guns are extremely useful to police, FBI, armed protection specialists, and others who carry guns all the time, concealed, not out and ready to use. There are many ways for a woman to have a gun ready when she needs it.

Having an appropriate "tool," knowing how to use it, and being willing to use it immeasurably enhances your chances of coming out alive in a confrontation where someone is trying to kill you.

The "tools" you choose are important, but there is no magic talisman that will ward off evil simply by displaying it. You have to know how to use your chosen tools and, if necessary, how to improvise if they are out of your possession.

Nancy Bittle, the founder of AWARE, said it best: "You should be armed with determination and intelligence, whether or not you have a physical weapon in your hand."

Let's take a look at some options.

❖ *"Empty-Handed" fighting*

There are basically two kinds of weaponless fighting, martial arts and full-contact self-defense specifically designed for women.

Martial arts are wonderful for exercise and confidence building, but they are sometimes overrated for self-defense. The martial arts forms that are fundamentally sports, with ranks, matches, and contests, take much time and effort to master and maintain. Generally police have found that other techniques are more effective "on the street." Any kind of training that requires you to "pull" strikes and kicks with a partner (so as not to hurt them) instead of hitting a person full force is not practical for self-defense. You will do in an emergency what you have done in practice; if you have practiced hitting people at less than full power, you cannot depend on your training to come through when you need it most.

There are some good martial arts programs if you look carefully. Try to find ones that feature techniques for very close quarter attacks like chokes, pins, and slams into a wall. Ground fighting is a particularly useful skill for women, who are often thrown to the ground during a fight. The program must involve full force blows against human assailants. One place to look for such programs in your area might be the National Women's Martial Arts Federation, on the web. (The web sites mentioned in this chapter appear in Appendix A.)

The alternative to martial arts is full-force, full-contact, padded-assailant fighting for women. This is never taught as a sport, but only as a set of effective defense techniques. One program that has spread widely in the last few years, particularly on college campuses, is RAD (Rape Aggression Defense). Another, that has been training women to fight effectively for nearly 20 years is Impact (in some places the name is Model Mugging); a list of studios nationwide is available on several web sites. Model Mugging was developed by a man, a martial artist, who knew a black-belt woman who was raped. Instead of blaming the woman for "allowing" the attack to occur, he thought deeply about the situation, and concluded that her training had failed her. He set out to develop a set of techniques that would be optimized to use women's strength (primarily in the legs rather than the arms) and to address the kinds of attacks that women often experience (such as grabs from the rear rather than attacks from the front). The result was Impact.

Look for training that involves realism, boundary setting, inner strength development, and ferocity development. Training should take place when you are in an adrenelated state so that you internalize the techniques better, and have confidence that they will work when you are under incredible stress.

It is impossible to underestimate the value of a course like this. If you already consider yourself "a fighter" based on your personality or your experience in sports, you will be able to learn defensive techniques that will surprise you.

If you consider yourself a wimp, someone who "could never fight back," a course like this will truly amaze you! You will be amazed at what you learn by finding your inner fighter and letting her out. You will amaze yourself, and you will amaze anyone foolish enough to try to force unwanted attentions on you.

A good basic self-defense course of this type should take somewhere in the range of 20-40 hours. We are not talking a lifelong or even year long commitment here, just a few concentrated hours to learn a few basic techniques, and how to use them full force in real fights against real assailants played by guys in padded suits. Some organizations offer less expensive refresher courses, to help you maintain your fighting skills.

Other ways to find this kind of training: ask at your local rape crisis centers, YWCA, community colleges and similar local organizations, or contact the American Women's Self-Defense Association (AWSDA) to find an instructor in your area.

❖ *Noisemakers*

Noisemakers include whistles, air horns, and battery-powered electronic "screamers". In general, these sorts of devices are over-rated, and may not provide the protection you need.

What do you expect of a noisemaker? That it will scare away your stalker if he approaches you? That someone will hear it and call the police?

If you are sure your stalker is mild-mannered and easily intimidated, then perhaps a blast of sound may send him running, but noise isn't going to deter someone intent on raping you, beating you, or killing you.

If you have made an advance pact with others in your community at work or around home that they will call the police if they hear your noisemaker, and if you have tested it under realistic conditions (will your neighbor hear it if she is in her kitchen? her bedroom?), then a noisemaker may have some value, but it absolutely cannot be depended upon to produce a reaction from a stranger who does not understand your plight.

Besides, using a noisemaker takes up at least one of your hands, which you could be using to better effect if you had a better defensive tool in it. If you must carry a noisemaker, be sure it isn't your only method of protection.

❖ *Pepper spray and other chemicals*

The primary chemicals on the market today are Pepper Spray (also known as Oleoresin Capsicum, or OC) and tear gas.

The original tear gas sprays were one of the first aerosol defensive sprays used by police, and used to be widely carried by ordinary citizens. Unfortunately, it is not very effective on the type of individuals that you may have to use it on, such as people who are under the influence of alcohol, drugs, in an emotional rage, or mentally unbalanced. Tear gas (and other kinds of defensive sprays) can also take quite a while to have an effect.

In most law enforcement applications, pepper spray has now replaced tear gas as the most effective less-than-lethal spray, and it is also the best defensive spray for people to carry. (Don't carry spray oven cleaner or other chemicals that would be dangerous if they happened to get on you by accident.)

Pepper spray contains the natural derivative of hot red peppers (capsaicin), which is concentrated and mixed with a carrier and a propellant to fill spray cans.

Unlike other sprays, pepper spray does not rely for its effectiveness on pain, but rather on the physical effects it causes. It makes the eyelids slam shut, temporarily but effectively blinding the attacker. It also causes severe breathing difficulties when inhaled, though it does not make the person stop breathing. People who are sprayed with it cough, choke, and gasp, and are frightened by being unable to breathe normally. Often, though not always, people drop to their knees or fall to the ground. In this condition, the will to fight is usually gone, as the attacker is disoriented, confused, and distracted.

If you spray someone with OC, aim for the face, where it will get into the eyes (even if he is wearing glasses), nose, and mouth, and on sensitive facial skin.

The effects are temporary, usually lasting 30 to 45 minutes.

It is effective on most people, including the mentally ill and those under the influence of drugs and alcohol. It also works on animals, such as dogs.

As part of becoming a certified instructor for OC spray, I had to be sprayed with it, so I understand the effects first hand! It is extremely unpleasant, but not life-threatening. I found the coughing and choking the most unpleasant and debilitating effect, though it wasn't much fun to be nearly blind either. After seeing its effect on other people, some of whom were highly trained fighters, I was completely convinced that pepper spray is a tool worth having!

This spray is an extremely effective general-purpose defense tool, but it is not a miracle product. Nothing is 100 percent effective, nor instantaneous. In particular, OC may not be effective on some violent, goal-oriented people and hardened attack dogs.

That means if someone is determined to kill you and has a gun, knife, or other contact weapon, they may be able to carry out their attack before the spray takes full effect, so OC would not be my defense tool of choice in such a situation. However, for use in less than life-threatening situations, this less-than-lethal product may be just the ticket.

The "heat" of these products is measured in Scoville Heat Units (SHU). Your average jalapeno pepper is around 5,000 SHUs; habaneros, the hottest peppers, are around 250,000 SHUs. When you buy OC, read the label carefully. The better brands will tell you the SHU rating. Look for a product with a SHU rating of 2 million or more!

The label should also tell you what the concentration of OC is in the can. The most effective concentration is 2% to 5%. Sometimes concentrations above 5% do not atomize well, and are therefore less effective. More is not always better!

Is OC spray legal? In most states, yes, but it does depend on your locality. In some places, anyone can buy it, in some places you need a license to purchase and possess it, in some places it is simply illegal. It used to be illegal to put it in checked baggage on a plane, but that has been changed. Don't try to carry it into the airplane's passenger compartment, however. That is not only highly illegal, but downright dangerous if it were to leak into the air during the flight.

As always, you need to verify the legality of any device or tool that you use.

Where can you buy defensive sprays? Again this depends on the laws in your area. It can vary from the hardware store or supermarket to a firearm store or a police supply store. They generally cost less than $20.

Don't get the tiny size designed to go on a keyring; it won't have enough oomph to be used outdoors if there is a breeze, and the range is a piddling 4-6 feet. Get the 2 oz size, which can be effective to about 12 feet, depending on the delivery system and the weather.

There are several types of spray delivery systems. The stream one, like a water pistol, is good if you plan to use the spray outdoors, in the wind. The cone-shaped spray, rather like hair spray, may be blown slightly off course by the wind, but is a better general-purpose choice. The fogger delivery system, which is just like it sounds, is designed to take care of multiple attackers. The sticky foam delivery system requires too much precision in placement. Since your stalker probably works alone, the cone spray is likely to be the best for you, unless you know you are likely to meet him outdoors.

Some companies are now marketing combinations of pepper spray and other active compounds. I don't recommend those, because there's not enough "street experience" to show whether these defensive cocktails are effective or just marketing hype. Simple pepper spray, on the other hand, has been around for decades, used successfully by many thousands of police officers and federal agencies such as the FBI.

It is handy to carry pepper spray in your purse or your coat pocket, but get in the habit of having it in your hand (even if your hand is in your pocket) at critical times, such as going to and from your car, or when waiting for public transportation. You need to be ready to deploy it instantly; if you have to search for it, you might as well have left it at home.

Speaking of home, some people buy several OC units and put one in their bedroom, one in their car, one in their purse…you get the idea. Wherever you keep it, remember to shake it about once a month because the ingredients do separate.

What if you spray someone with it, and you get some of the spray on yourself? I've had this happen too, and can attest that going through OC already in the air is much less awful than being sprayed with it directly. Besides, if you can move away from the spray as you use it, you can greatly reduce the chance that you will be exposed to any of it. That's one of the things you can learn in training.

If you intend to buy a defensive spray, you should try to find a class (generally just 2-3 hours) that trains you how to use it. Police carry OC spray, but generally they must take a class first. You should have similar training, perhaps from an instructor recommended by your local police department, to learn how to effectively control a situation, and the difference between effective and ineffective application (too near, too far, or too much spray used, etc.). You need to practice short bursts, usually less than one second. Proper use of pepper spray is not like hosing down a bug with a can of Raid!

The class should cover such things as legal issues, what the various differences in concentration, canister size, valve type, etc. mean in terms of how it should be used, how to carry it, how to use it, what the effective range is, the effects of wind direction, why you should report the incident to the police if you have to use it, what to do if you get some on you, how long the effects might last and what sorts of people and situations it might or might not be effective for. The best training will also include practice with "training units," spray cans just like the one you will carry, but filled with an inert, non-irritating substance, so you can get the feel of how the spray can operates and how to spray and move so that you are not exposed to the spray.

Pepper spray is easy-to-use, effective, inexpensive, and useful in a wide range of situations. The FBI has tested it extensively, and approved its use as a non-lethal tool for controlling aggressive people. Doesn't it sound like something you want to have on hand?

❖ *Persuader / Kubotan*

A Persuader (also called a Kubotan, or other trade names) is a slender plastic stick 5 1/2 inches long and 5/8 inch in diameter, with a key ring attached to a swivel on one end. It has no other actions or features, but it is amazingly effective for doing strikes, blocking someone trying to hit you, and escaping from someone who has grabbed you.

They generally come with either ridges or grooves; the ridged ones are quite a bit more effective and less likely to slip in your hand.

You can use the Persuader as a striking tool, holding the plastic rod in your hand and swinging the keys on the swivel. Or you can hold the Persuader in any of several different grips, and use either blunt end (or the sharp edge of the blunt end) against vulnerable areas such as the eyes, throat, groin, or back of the hands.

Once you know the basics of fighting with a Persuader, which means knowing various pressure points on an assailant's body, it is easy to improvise when you don't have one with you, by using a pen, a table knife, a small flashlight, or your own fingers.

Many police officers carry them, for convenience in "persuading" a recalcitrant person into custody without resorting to a larger, more forceful option, such as a baton.

Until recently, they were legal to take on airplanes, but this has changed. Enforcement may vary depending on your airline and the particular security people you encounter. To be sure your trip isn't interrupted by a lengthy discussion with the security folks, you might want to put your Persuader in your checked baggage.

You can buy Kubotans and Persuaders (generally under $10) at police supply stores, some firearms stores, some martial arts supply stores, and some mail order sources and web sites.

Like any self defense tool, you need training in how to use it.

To find a certified instructor, you might have to inquire of your local police department who certifies police, and then find out if that person will teach a class that is specially adapted for civilians. The class should emphasize strikes and releases that allow you to escape, NOT the standard police training that focuses on control holds that keep you close to the attacker in order to lead to handcuffing.

❖ *Knives*

A knife can be an excellent defense tool, but it can be difficult to distinguish between good and bad knives and equally difficult to distinguish between good and bad knife fighting instructors in today's climate of obsessive macho.

Never have switchblades (knives that spring open) or gravity knives (that fall open); they are illegal and dangerous.

Never depend for your life on a simple kitchen knife, or a little "pen knife," Boy Scout knife, or Swiss Army knife—all of these knives may break, may close on your own finger, may be inadequately sharp, or may allow your hand to slip from the handle onto the blade when you thrust hard with slippery, sweaty hands.

Spyderco, Benchmade, and Cold Steel are some of the companies that make good folding knives of the sort that are often carried by police and other emergency responders. You can buy these knives at many sporting goods stores, police supply stores, or similar outlets, or on the Internet.

Basically, a good defensive knife should be large enough to fit comfortably in the palm of your hand when closed, and its blade should be well within the legal limit in your state when it is open.

It should be easy to open the knife and lock the blade with one hand, after a minute or two of practice. The handle should not be smooth, lest the knife slip in your hand. Most modern defensive knives come with a clip so you can fasten it in a pocket, on a waistband, or somewhere in a purse so that you can always reach to the same place whenever you need to draw the knife.

When searching for an instructor, stay away from martial artists who teach a knife course on the side. Unless you have a lot of evidence to the contrary, they are likely to be more show than substance. Look for someone who teaches a variety of different defensive methods, and whose emphasis is on simple, effective techniques.

❖ *Stun guns*

A stun gun is a small, hand-held, battery-powered electrical device that is capable of producing an electric shock with two probes that must be held against the attacker's body.

Unfortunately, people who carry stun guns often believe that they will instantly incapacitate an attacker. Nothing could be further from the truth. I've been subjected to the effects of a stun gun in training, and not only I, but every other member of the class, stayed on our feet and were able to react with defensive techniques.

Like a Persuader, a stun gun is a contact weapon that cannot be deployed at a distance. In fact, to use it most effectively, you need to hold it in close contact with skin or a lightly clothed area for at least 3 seconds. That's an awfully long time.

Heavy clothing, such as a leather jacket, can adversely affect its performance. Some people are also quite impervious to the shock, due to their mental state, some innate physical characteristic, or because they have built up a tolerance.

Stun guns cost $50 to around $200, and may be purchased in gun stores or from safety product companies. They are illegal in many states, so check into your local laws (and the laws of any place you may travel).

If you decide to get one, you might want to test it on your arm or leg so you understand its properties.

❖ *Firearms*

Guns are a sensitive topic for many people, but one that we have to address in this book. Not to do so would leave you without a very important option.

Let me take a moment here for a personal aside. I have been shooting for more than 15 years, specializing in the use of firearms for defensive purposes. I have been trained by police and former members of the military; I have shot in tactical competitions against police and people from federal law enforcement agencies, I have published more than a hundred articles about defense in *Women & Guns* magazine, and have won awards for writing and teaching about the defensive uses of firearms. I am a certified firearms instructor. And most important of all, I never picked up a gun until well into adulthood, so I started out with all the fears and objections to firearms that may be in your mind, too.

If you have never learned how to handle a gun, you probably think of a gun as something like a bomb—something very dangerous that could go off at any time, something that kills people, something that only police experts should handle. But to me, and to many of the women I've taught, *a gun is like a fire extinguisher*—something I hope I never have to use, but a life-saving piece of emergency equipment that I can use to keep myself, and my family, alive until the professionals can get on the scene to take over.

If you decide to get a gun, you are not alone. Up to 17% of stalking victims arm themselves. That is 1 in 6.

First and foremost, do not get a gun unless you also get adequate, appropriate training in how to use it. You will need three kinds of training, which may come in the same class, or may be in different courses: training in handling a gun safely, training in how to shoot accurately, and training in the defensive use of firearms. The total time involved should be a minimum of about 40 hours.

For basic safety and "how to shoot" training, the instructor should provide a selection of firearms, so you don't have to buy and bring your own. This lets you try a number of different kinds of guns before deciding what (or whether) to purchase. Some guns that are comfortable to hold are very uncomfortable to shoot, and vice versa, so you cannot adequately choose a gun without having fired a similar make and model.

You should get as much shooting instruction as possible before making the decision whether you want to buy a gun or not. You wouldn't buy a horse after just one riding lesson, would you?

It takes time to get over the natural fear of guns that is harbored by most adults who have never used them, and it also takes time to understand the realities and responsibilities of gun ownership. If you aren't ready to take on the responsibility, don't buy a gun (yet), but do get training anyway.

to take on the responsibility, don't buy a gun (yet), but do get training anyway.

➤ When might you need a gun?

The answer to that question is short and bleak: when your stalker decides to kill you.

Stalkers who plan murder-suicides do so either as part of a deranged plan to be together in the hereafter, or because a controlling man cannot deal with the loss of the woman he had dominated and thinks this is the only way to end his pain.

Unfortunately, there are many, many stories that bear this out. One was reported by Ellen Sorokin in her *Washington Times* article on the limitations of anti-stalking laws: "Janice Michelle Lancaster, of Faulker, had a protective order. Only five days before her death on Jan 3, 2000, the Charles County District Court officially notified her 36-year old estranged husband, a man who was her high school sweetheart, he was not to come near her. The four-page document was all she was armed with when James Lancaster crept into her home on Popes Creed Road at 6 a.m. and hunted her down with a loaded shotgun."

This kind of extreme situation happens to a very small percentage of stalking victims, but it does happen. If it happens to you, even if you summon the police as soon as possible, you will have to keep yourself alive until the police get there, which will be 3 to 5 minutes under the best of circumstances, possibly much longer. I don't know any tool other than a gun that will reliably keep you alive in that situation.

➤ Common fears about guns

If you are a reasonable, mature, responsible adult who has never had anything to do with guns, the thought of using one to defend yourself immediately raises many concerns. Here are some of the common ones…

Fear you won't be able to hit him. The antidote to this fear is having the skill to use a gun effectively. Your training will soon show you what size targets you can hit effectively, at what distances, and under what conditions.

Fear of having the gun being taken away and used against you. This is a plaintive cry often heard from well-meaning people who are quite wrong. I have heard of a number of cases where a stalker was shot before he could kill his victim. I have heard of cases where the stalker was frightened into stopping his activities when he was threatened with a gun. But I have never found a single verifiable case where a properly trained private citizen had a gun taken away from her in a situation where she needed it for her own defense.

Fundamentally, if you are willing to shoot the person who is trying to kill you, you can shoot him before he can take the gun away. He will most likely know this, and will not even try to get at your gun. But if he does try, you have the power to stop him!

Fear that you may freeze instead of shooting when it is necessary. Why do so many women fear that they will react this way? If you have had the experience of being so startled by someone or something that you gasp and remain motionless for a moment, you might think that that motionless state will continue if you ever experience a full-fledged attack.

Dr. Alexis Artwohl, a psychologist who interviews many police officers who have been through deadly force confrontations, compiles statistics on the perceptual distortions that occur during those incidents. According to her studies, only 12% of people experience a feeling of temporary paralysis during an attack, and even for them, it is temporary.

The more you practice how to react in a situation, the more confident you will become that you could handle a tough situation without freezing.

Fear that you may make a mistake in judgment and shoot the wrong person. Many people are tortured by the question, "Will I make the right decision?" Just the fact that you formulate that question, and worry about it, shows that you are a responsible person who is concerned about doing the right thing.

Perhaps a few facts will help to reduce that level of tortured self-doubt to something bearable. The following comes from Skip Gochenour, the director of the American Tactical Shooting Association.

"Each year in the United States armed citizens kill 2.5 to 3 times as many felons in lawful and justifiable use of force encounters as do the police. In these incidents, police kill innocent parties about 11% of the time. Armed citizens make the same mistake about 2% of the time. Police mistakenly kill innocent citizens five times more often than armed citizens do in justifiable use of force incidents."

Think hard about that. Armed private citizens make many fewer mistakes than police when it comes to shooting people! Why? Well, for one thing, a private citizen is right there on the spot from the beginning to the end of an attack; she (or he) has a much easier job of sorting out the good guy (self) from the bad guys than do the police, who arrive in the middle of a scene full of participants they have never seen before.

Fear that the gun will not be available when you need it. If it is legal for you to carry a gun in public, you can do so. There are now enough different kinds of holster options available so that it is possible for most women to have a gun within reach virtually all the time. Don't fall for the line that guns are useless because you might be attacked suddenly; if that were true, police would not carry guns.

Fear of a tragic accident. Again, training is the answer here. It is easy to learn how to handle a gun safely, how to store it safely, and how to keep it out of unauthorized hands.

A trigger lock should NEVER be used on a loaded gun, but there are other ways of locking a loaded gun so that it is accessible to the authorized user but not to other people. For example, you can get a lockbox, which is a small metal safe designed to hold a loaded gun. The best ones have push-button locks that allow you to set the combination you want, and that (unlike dial locks on traditional safes and padlocks) can be operated by touch, in the dark, even when your hands are shaking badly.

Many people believe, falsely, that guns are exceedingly dangerous to their owners. This belief is fostered by misleading factoids that get a lot of press, but that aren't true, and are not relevant to a situation where a stalking victim is preparing to defend her life, if necessary, from someone who may try to murder her. In those extreme circumstances, a gun can be a lifeline!

Fear of what other people will say. It is natural to be concerned about what other people think of us, and comments such as "You're getting a gun—you must be paranoid!" or "What are you, some kind of vigilante?" can cut deep. Remember that your friends, even your family, don't always understand the danger you are in. Having a few calm responses prepared, such as "I'm not paranoid, just careful," and "Vigilante? No, of course not. That's against the law. But self-defense is legal." may help you weather the storm of protest you may experience. Another approach is to be very low key, and not let people know you are armed.

➤ Why do police carry guns?

That's a serious question. If police always had time to call for backup, guns could be kept at the police station and brought out "only when needed." If less-lethal options such as pepper spray, batons, and hands-on techniques were always sufficient to control any situation, police would carry them instead of guns. But they don't. Police carry guns in addition to all the other equipment and training they have available. Why? Because there are some situations in which nothing else will work, when the threat to the police officer or some person is so violent, and so immediate, that nothing less than lethal force will save an innocent life.

If a police officer happened to be standing around when your deranged stalker started stabbing you with a knife in a murderous frenzy, wouldn't you expect the officer to do whatever was necessary to save your life, including shooting the stalker before he could stab you again?

If you decide to get a firearm, and the training to go with it, it should be for the same reasons, as a last-ditch tool for use in a life-or-death confrontation when there is no possibility of being saved by someone else, so you have to save your life yourself. This is the only valid reason for getting a gun.

When I was writing this section, I heard the news that a doctor in Massachusetts had just murdered his estranged wife, shooting her in her home, in the presence of several of their children. With immense sadness, I try to imagine what she could have done in that situation to save her life; I can't think of anything that would have given her a fighting chance, other than having her own gun.

Imagine for a moment that an armed police officer had been present in that woman's home when her husband tried to kill her. If there was no other way to save that woman's life, the officer would have to shoot the husband. If you believe, as I do, and as most people do, that the police officer would have been justified in using lethal force to save that woman from being murdered, then the natural corollary is that, in the absence of a police officer, the woman herself would have been justified in using lethal force in that same situation, to save her own life and her children's lives as well.

➤ Guns and stalking

A recent study published in a journal produced by the national Centers for Disease Control and Prevention looked carefully at stalking in the state of Louisiana, and turned up some unexpected results. According to that report, 70% of those stalked reported changing their usual behavior to discourage the stalking; 36% said they had moved their homes; 11% said they got a restraining order…and 11% said they obtained a gun for protection. A different study found 17% of stalking victims armed themselves.

The pros and cons of restraining orders are discussed elsewhere in this book, but would you have expected that as many stalking victims are getting guns as restraining orders?

If you make the decision to get a firearm, you won't be alone. Many people who experience the extreme danger of being the focus of a potentially murderous stalker decide that it is better to have a gun and not need it, than to need a gun, and not have it.

➤ Practical and legal issues

A new, good quality firearm will cost from a few hundred dollars to around a thousand (in general, revolvers will cost less than semi-automatic handguns). Add money for training, ammunition to practice with, a safe storage system, and licensing fees, and you can easily spend double your gun cost on these additional items.

Don't let the cost deter you. If you can't afford a new gun, reliable second-hand ones are widely available. Many training organizations will work with you to get you the training and equipment that you need, if you explain the danger you are in.

Many women who can legally carry a gun in public choose to carry their gun in their purse; this is much slower to access than a gun holstered somewhere on your body. Be prepared to make some changes in your wardrobe if you carry a gun public. Tight-fitting clothing is generally incompatible with wearing a holstered gun. There are many, many more ways to conceal a gun than you would think. *Women&Guns* magazine has frequent reviews of various products and methods of concealed carry.

In the last few years, many states have revised their firearms laws, so that now most states allow people to own firearms in their homes, and a majority of states now allow properly licensed people to carry a concealed firearm in public.

Laws regarding where you can, and can't, have a gun (such as whether you can leave a gun locked in the glove compartment of your car, for example), vary greatly from place to place. You should look for information about laws from several sources, such as the police licensing authority (not just any police officer), people in the firearms sales or training business, and lawyers who have had considerable experience with firearms issues (most lawyers have very little experience in this area).

➤ Training sources

Buying a gun without getting training is like buying a bathing suit without taking swimming lessons; you may look and feel fine, but you don't know how to save your own life in an emergency. Get training!

Regardless of what you think of the National Rifle Association (NRA), they have excellent introductory courses for firearm safety and marksmanship, and they have instructors all over the country. Check out their training web site.

A number of firearms makers, including SIGarms and Smith&Wesson have established academies with courses for responsible private citizens.

There are also many excellent private shooting schools around the country where you can get the instruction you need to be able to protect your life, responsibly. There are several lists of such schools on the web.

Be sure to find training, at least at first, which does not require you to already own a gun. I hate to make generalizations about how women and men regard firearms differently, but I'll risk making just one, based on years of experience teaching and observing both sexes. Men tend to decide that they would use a gun if necessary, then they buy one, then they get training. Women tend to follow the *opposite* path: they tend to get training, then some of them decide to buy a gun, and only then (often after more training) do some of them decide that they could use the gun defensively if necessary.

Don't get a gun until you are ready. Do get training, even if you hate guns and think you could never use one.

How much training do you need? I've seen novices turn into people I'd be glad to have by my side in an armed confrontation in about 40 hours of intensive training from top quality instructors. You should probably plan on a total of 40-80 hours of instruction, and, you should plan to practice about once a month if possible.

➤ Have other defenses

Finally, if you have a gun for defense, it must not be your only defense!

Remember that police who carry guns also carry OC spray, a radio, and an impact weapon or two. You should have training in at least one other less-lethal method of defense, so that you can choose the most appropriate response to a situation, and you should always try to have a means of communication such as a cellphone with you, to call for help if there is time to do so.

➤ A success story

Joanne Carroll had a lot of trouble with her ex-husband, Michael. He had run her car off the road; he dragged her, pregnant, from a moving car;

and twice he threatened to cut off her son's tongue. Even after she left him, he continued to beat, chase, and stalk her.

Joanne took a number of steps to protect herself and her family. She got self-defense training, obtained a license to carry firearms, and got a 9mm semi-automatic to carry and a shotgun to use at home.

In June 1996, she was driving home when Michael drove up behind her, and tried to force her car off the road. She reached for her gun, and held it to the car window where he could see it clearly. For the first time ever, Michael was intimidated. He drove away without trying further to hurt her.

Michael was quickly convicted of assault with a dangerous weapon (his car) and violating a restraining order, charges that resulted in a five year sentence, giving Joanne an opportunity to further extend her plans to protect her family when he next gets out of prison.

It may be surprising, but this is a very typical defensive use of a firearm: no shots are fired, but the woman is safe because she had a gun and was prepared to use it if necessary.

❖ Defensive driving

You don't normally think of your car as a defensive tool, but it can be. Think of how much time you spend in your car—isn't it worth some special effort to learn to protect yourself when you are in it?

Defensive driving is not what you learned in your high school driving class. Instead, it means the techniques that specialists teach to police and to people providing protective services.

There are a number of excellent "driving academies" where you can learn a phenomenal amount about how to take care of yourself in a car, such as the Scotti School, the Bob Bondurant School of High Performance Driving, and BSR Inc. Most of them have web sites. These schools teach racing driving, but many of them have defensive driving courses as well. There is probably a good driving school near you; to find it, ask around for someone who trains police or other emergency personnel.

If you can't take a driving class, at least read the book *Drive to Survive* by Curt Rich. It is a good starting point; this book will show you how to adjust your mirrors so there is no blind spot, how to spot someone following you and what to do about it. The chapter on kidnapping and carjacking also has much valuable information for any woman who is being stalked.

❖ *Improvised weapons*

You can turn virtually anything into a self-defense tool under sufficient duress. You should not count on "found weapons" instead of training with "real" weapons, but if you don't have a "real" tool when you need one, you should creatively use whatever is at hand.

Here are just a few of the things that you can turn into devastating, surprisingly effective weapons:

- pen or pencil
- scissors
- lamp
- metal nail file
- book (shove a corner into a tender area, such as genitals or abdomen)
- tightly rolled magazine or newspaper (ditto)
- purse
- keys (hold in your fist in the usual way, not with keys sticking out between your fingers)

- umbrella
- kitchen knife
- pots or pans
- broom handle
- cane
- a belt (take it off, hold wrap one end around your hand and swing the other at his eyes and groin, HARD)
- …you get the idea!

You can create a club-substitute dropping any small, dense object (a cake of soap, a heavy ashtray, a paperweight, a TV remote control,…) into a sock. This will let you repeatedly swing HARD at an assailant, and is much more effective than trying to throw those objects at him. Don't have a sock? You can also use the toe of pantyhose, or a shirt sleeve with a knot tied near the cuff.

Look around you now. What could you use to help protect yourself with if necessary?

Even with improvised weapons, you should practice in advance. Grab a book or rolled up newspaper and try some strikes in the air. Try swinging soap-in-a-sock, or a can of tuna in a blouse sleeve, so that you get the idea of it firmly in your mind, and in your muscle memory. Then you will be more likely to think of these things when you need them.

Whatever improvised weapon you use, employ it with extreme vigor!

❖ *Diversify your safety portfolio*

Just as diversifying your financial portfolio is the best way to take care of your financial assets, one of the best ways to take care of yourself is to diversify your safety skills.

Get training in several types of self-defense and/or several types of defensive tools, and then decide which ones you want to bet your life on.

Notice that I did NOT say you should choose a particular weapon first, and then learn to use it. You cannot make intelligent, informed decisions about your own safety until you acquire some of the skill to utilize a particular weapon. This goes for knives, dogs, pepper spray, guns, and other weapons as well.

Interlude 4: What would you do?

You are a manager in a medium-sized high tech company. You hire a new employee for a fairly high-level position, but right from the start there are problems. He can't seem to fit in and get the work done, and the other employees constantly clash with him.

After a few months of trying to be boss, mentor, and mediator, you have had enough. You do some groundwork with your Human Resources officer to document the seriousness of the problems. You call him into your office (with the HR rep), and gently break the news that he will have to leave.

He goes ballistic, calling you names and swearing that he will "make the whole company sorry" for firing him. The look on his face frightens you deeply, though you try not to show it, and you are relieved when he runs out of the office.

That night, you receive three hangup calls at home, more than you have ever gotten before.

The next morning, when you walk into your office, you find a round of rifle ammunition on the floor just inside the door, and your heart stops beating for a few seconds as you remember his enraged face. But there is no way to prove it came from him.

What would you do?

Again, this situation calls for a coordinated effort to ensure your safety. Informing Human Resources and the police is undoubtedly a good idea, though there is not much they can actually do at this point.

Maybe your company will retain an expert in workplace violence to help evaluate the situation.

Meantime, you should be taking a great many precautions, starting with increased awareness at all times, particularly when you are coming and going from work. Is he watching you? Is he following you? This would be a good time to brush up on your self-defense techniques and tools (or to learn them, if you need to). Most disgruntled employees cool down, and don't become violent, so you need to be especially viligant right away, when the danger is highest.

The implied threat of the ammunition, and (assuming he was the hangup caller) the fact that he knows your home telephone number (and probably knows or can find out where you live) is going to be very frightening. That's why he did those things, to upset you. Your company can do a lot to help ensure your safety while you are on the premises. Co-workers who know he should not be in the building can instantly report if they see him, for example. But you are on your own once you leave work, and you should be very, very cautious.

11 Interacting with "The System"

As a stalking victim, you will have a lot of "finding out" to do. Because laws, policies, procedures, and people differ widely from one location to another, it is almost impossible to put in one book all the things you will need to know and do to have a good result from "the system" of legal and other organizations.

To "find out" something mentioned in this chapter, you might start by asking the police officers you interact with. You could also talk to a lawyer or Legal Aid, people in a local women's shelter, or you could call the prosecutor's office that would handle your case. You can find the prosecutor in the state listing section of the yellow pages.

In some places, lawyers, the police, prosecutors, and social agencies are knowledgeable about stalking, and well coordinated so that they operate almost as a team, and can tell you exactly what to expect from "the system" in terms of protection for you and arrest for your stalker. I've met stalking victims who were extremely pleased with the response they got from the police and other agencies.

In some other places, you may know more about stalking than some of the people who are supposed to help you, and you will have to help educate them. There are some stalking victims who are very unhappy with the response "the system" is making to their situation.

One stalking victim says: "The various pieces of the judicial system and law enforcement are not always well versed about the seriousness of stalking, nor are they synchronized as to the prosecution and/or the enforcement of the stalking laws. It is possible to get various answers to the same questions depending upon who you talk to. It is imperative NOT to assume that these individuals have all the answers or necessarily the right ones.

The individual [being stalked] MUST take responsibility for her own safety and well-being, first and foremost. First, she must ask questions. If she gets conflicting information, she shouldn't make assumptions that everything will be taken care of or straightened out because these 'professionals' know what they're doing. It is far too easy for people or cases to drop through the cracks and there are far too many that do."

So, be prepared to ask lots and lots of questions. Ask everyone questions like: "What should I do now?" "How long will that take?" "Will you notify me? How?" "How many cases similar to mine have you handled before?" "What criteria have to be met in order for you to take action regarding my situation?" "Who else should I talk to?" "Who has dealt with stalking cases—can I talk to him/her?"

Ask, and ask, and ask....

❖ *Police*

Report each and every stalking incident, even if the police seem uninterested. You may need to explicitly request that your calls be logged, or a report made.

In most places, police officers are required to make written reports when citizens request them, so make an explicit request that the officers make a report whenever you contact them about the stalking. Find out your case number, if one is assigned. Get the names and badge numbers of any police officers you talk to about the stalking.

Find out if the police will file all your reports under the same case number.

Ask for copies of all the police reports that you make.

Try to see to it that each police report references the one(s) that have come before. Otherwise, someone reviewing a report will have no way of knowing that it is part of a pattern.

Find out if the police will assign a single detective to your case. If so, call him or her from time to time to get an update on your case. If not, you should call others in the police department who have dealt with your incidents.

If you report incidents to different law enforcement agencies, whether in the same geographic location or different ones, try to make sure that they are each aware of the other's reports.

Whenever you interact with police, try to have evidence with you to show them. Also, have a written (preferably typed) summary of your situation—a copy you can give them.

Be aware that just because a warrant has been issued for someone's arrest, that doesn't mean that the police will immediately be dispatched to pick him up. In some parts of the country, police are so overloaded that warrants pile up, particularly for offenses that are considered "less serious." It recently came to light that Charles Jaynes, the man who kidnapped and murdered a 10-year old Boston boy, had 75 active warrants out for his arrest before he committed murder. An investigative reporter found that Massachusetts has around half a million unserved warrants, Florida has 300,000, and California has 2.5 million! You may have to keep pushing to find out whether a warrant in your case has actually been served.

In many areas, there are not good computerized records accessible to police in a timely manner. This includes, particularly, information about restraining orders and violations thereof. Kristen Lardner was murdered by her boyfriend, Michael Cartier, while he was on probation for attacking a previous girlfriend, and while there was a warrant out for his arrest. Kristen filed for two civil court restraining orders. The courts were unaware of the details of Michael's criminal history, and the resulting orders were ineffective. He followed Kristen and shot her to death in the middle of a Boston street. So, don't assume that different parts of "the system" will communicate about your problem—be sure to inform the police departments where you live and where you work about your situation, and about any restraining orders you have.

You might want to have a supportive friend or family member along whenever you have a meeting with police, prosecutors, attorneys, or other such folk. Two sets of eyes and ears will be better than one. You might ask your companion to take notes, so you will be free to concentrate on the conversation you are having. If you cannot take a friend along, take a tape recorder, and remember to ask for permission to use it.

❖ Witnesses

If there are witnesses to any stalking incidents, talk to them about whether they will testify in court if need be. Remember your stalking log? Put the witness's responses about testifying there, and get their address and/or phone number.

If your family, co-workers and friends are occasionally witnesses to your stalking, or if the stalker has any interactions with them directly, ask them to write their own logs of these events as well.

❖ Lawyers

You might want to have an attorney send a registered letter to the stalker that he must stop harassing you immediately, and threatening him with arrest if he continues to bother you. This is unlikely to have much of an effect on a seriously disturbed stalker, but it might intimidate some people who have a lot to lose. It might also provide proof to a court later that you really did want him to stop, and that he knew it. But it might also make the stalker more angry, so discuss this step carefully with a number of experts before taking it.

Talk to a lawyer about what exactly constitutes stalking or related crimes in your state, and what it takes to get a prosecutor to bring a case to trial.

Find out whether a first time stalking offense is a felony or a misdemeanor in your state, as this will indicate how seriously the legal system perceives it.

❖ *Prosecutors*

Once the police investigator thinks that there is "probable cause" to arrest the stalker, he or she must request the prosecutor to authorize a warrant for the arrest. In some cases, however, the police or prosecutor may feel that not enough evidence exists, or that the pattern of behavior is not sufficiently 'criminal' to result in a successful prosecution. If the investigating officer assigned to your case does not seek an arrest warrant, you may be able to contact the prosecutor directly to discuss your situation and request the warrant.

Crime victims can often take an active part in the bail-setting process. Try to speak with the prosecuting attorney at the time of arraignment, to insist that a high bail be set. Also try to get the prosecutor to ask the court for a "no-contact" order—in some places it is called a "stay away" order—as a condition of pretrial release. This is stronger than a simple restraining order, because violating it means that he can be immediately jailed without release until the trial. If the stalker has to be released, ask whether he can be required to wear a bracelet or wristband that keeps the authorities informed of his location.

Monitoring systems are not a panacea, however. Some courts and law enforcement officers have a poor understanding of the potential danger of stalkers. Melita Schaum reports that "Illinois victim Dawn Wilson, stalked and attacked by her ex-husband, was horrified to learn of his release after he had accrued 223 technical violations of the electronic monitoring system he had been placed on to ensure that he stay away from her."

Ask to be notified of your stalker's potential release on parole; that is, before the parole hearing takes place, if you are allowed to provide information to the parole board.

Ensure that every police or legal interaction with the stalker has an outcome that he perceives as negative. Easy bail, light sentences, and unsupervised release of stalkers are generally ineffective, and send the message that the "system" won't react strongly enough to prevent him from continuing his harassment.

Find out if you are entitled to the services of a victim advocate. Most states have them, their services are free, and they will help you negotiate the maze of the legal system.

Find out whether your state allows stalking victims to pursue restitution against a stalker in civil court. (I know of a woman, a financial consultant, who sued her stalker, a former client, for monetary damages, and the stalking ceased, at least temporarily.) You may be able to sue for emotional, physical, or financial damages. You may be able to recover the cost of property damaged by the stalker, or the cost of your medical expenses or even the cost of therapy made necessary by the stalking.

You may be able to influence what the police look for if they get a search warrant for your stalker. At the 1999 Threat Assessment Conference, Assistant DA Rhonda Saunders said that some good things to ask for in a search warrant are:

- weapons

- computer and related equipment
- surveillance devices or catalogs
- maps
- letters
- photos
- Rolodex or other address or phone list
- phone records
- objects belonging to you, the victim.

❖ *Newspapers, TV, radio, politicians*

If you are comfortable doing so, approach local media, newspapers, local magazines, TV broadcasters, cable TV, radio, and so on. You can write to the host or producer, or call the station and ask to talk to the show's producer. The producer, not the host, is usually the one who decides what people and subjects appear on the show.

The stations that have public service features or public advocacy programs may want your story.

If you feel uncomfortable in front of a camera or microphone, or are afraid that appearing would endanger you, you can still make yourself available for interviews by asking the producer to disguise your voice or appearance for safety.

Radio talk shows can be a popular, and effective, way to get your information broadcast, and all you have to do to get on is to call the number they mention on the air.

If you are comfortable doing so, talk to local politicians—your state senators and representatives. Tell your story, and ask for their help in getting the police to intervene, getting the prosecutor to prosecute, or getting the laws changed. Don't worry if you are interviewed by a staff member instead of the politician him/herself. The staff of most political figures are knowledgeable, helpful people who are genuinely powerful in shaping their boss' opinions and actions.

12 Questions Stalking Victims Ask

❖ *"What else can I do?"*

• Share with others in the same situation

Join a stalking victims' support group. Not only is it wonderful to share experiences with people who really understand, but this is a good place to learn about and share safety tips.

• Have your stalker monitored

Ineffective monitoring of stalkers is a common complaint from stalking victims. The technology now exists for stalkers to wear monitoring bracelets that allow their positions to be precisely known. Fight for this to be used on your stalker if he is released on bail, or on parole. If you are told that the equipment is not available, ask if they would use it if it were, and consider having a fund-raiser to raise money to buy it for your locale.

• Know your weapons

If you carry any defensive devices, such as a Persuader, stun gun, OC spray, or a firearm, be sure you understand the uses and limitations of each one. Get training!

• Change your habits

This is terribly important, but some women do not want to do it, because it acknowledges the "effect" that the stalker has on them. It is better (and safer) to acknowledge that effect, and take steps to deal with it. It is foolish, ineffective, and simply untrue to pretend that your life has not been changed by the stalker, or that you don't need to do anything differently to be safe. One stalking victim says that as a result of the changes she has made in her life, she is "no longer afraid, just careful."

Shop someplace new.

Change your hair style, or find a new hairdresser. Buy a wig.

Change your clothing style and accessories.

• Find local resources

Find out the location of your local crime victim's resource center, women's shelter, legal aid office, stalking victims support group and other local organizations. A local library, police station, phone book, or town hall are all a good starting points for this information.

Check out your local library for books on stalking, and on self-protection.

• Stick with your friends

Always assume that your stalker may be watching you, and prepare accordingly; do more things with friends, fewer things alone.

Always keep enough cash on hand to get by for a day or so, in case you can't get to an ATM.

When you go out, try to go with a friend who understands your situation. Try not to go out alone at night.

Be sure that someone knows where you are at all times, and when you expect to be home. If you cannot leave this information with a specific person, write it down and put it in a consistent place, so that it can easily be found if you go missing.

• Refuse deliveries

Refuse flowers or other deliveries unless you are sure you know who they are from. Tell the florist to take the flowers to a local hospital as a donation. Don't take them there yourself, it may look to the stalker as if you accepted them.

• Make a "wanted" poster for your stalker

Prepare a short handout about your stalker, with a picture if one is available. It should include all of the following, if you know them: a physical description of him, a description of his car and its license number, a description of what kinds of things he has been doing that constitute stalking, mention of any restraining orders you have, and what to do if someone notices him near you, trying to reach you, or trying to find out information about you (for example call the police, or call company security). Have copies of these made so you can hand them out to neighbors, friends, co-workers, and others.

• Don't retaliate

Refrain from retaliation of any kind. Do not follow him, vandalize his car or home, or encourage anyone else to do such things. Doing so could place you in danger, physically, and legally, and could be used against you in any legal action against the stalker. Do not joke or talk about wanting to kill the stalker; you may have to kill him someday, and those words could be used against you in court.

- ## Set false leads

Directly confronting your stalker is NOT a safe idea, but you might want to outwit him without confrontation by setting false leads for him to follow, such as a post office box you don't really use, or a phone in your name that he can discover, but that isn't your real phone.

- ## Be aware of potential changes to laws that affect you

In some states there are court challenges to stalking laws, to ensure that labor picketers or other lawful demonstrators do not find themselves changed with stalking. The legitimate conduct of some businesses, like news reporting or a private detective agency, may require some activities such as surveillance that would normally be considered stalking, so they may be exempt. Should paparazzi be chargeable under stalking laws, or be exempt? If you hear that the stalking laws in your state are undergoing changes or court challenges, you might want to make your opinions known, to be sure that you remain protected.

❖ *"Should I hire a bodyguard?"*

They are not called bodyguards any more, they are now personal protection specialists, and they are generally quite expensive.

Before you spend money on one, figure out exactly what you need. Do you need an escort to a court appearance for a few hours, or do you need an escort to and from work every day? Do you need someone to be a visual deterrent to an attacker, or someone who is trained, equipped, and prepared to intervene to save your life if you are attacked?

Be absolutely sure that the person you are hiring has specific personal protection training, not just prior law enforcement experience, and ask for references from other stalking victims.

❖ *"Should I get a restraining order?"*

There is no issue more controversial than this. Even the experts disagree.

In some places, a Restraining Order (RO) is called an Order of Protection. In many places, there are similar, but not identical, orders with other names, so be sure you talk with some local experts about what is available in your area, and exactly what they mean.

Let's look at the pros and cons.

Pro: ROs can be effective as a deterrent, and essential as an enforcement tool against the stalker. In particular, most stalkers will try to defend themselves in court by saying, "I didn't mean to scare her," since intent to put you in fear is part of the requirement of stalking. But if you took a RO out against him, it is much harder for him to claim that he "didn't know" he was frightening you, or didn't mean to scare you when he violated the RO.

Con: ROs aggravate the stalker and may cause him to escalate his efforts, even resort to violence. ROs are pieces of paper that offer no real protection. Inadequate follow-up when ROs are violated may further embolden the stalker.

Gavin de Becker believes ROs may be as likely to provoke an obsessed individual as to restrain him. DeBecker says, "Cases which escalated to violence have one factor in common alarmingly often: INTERVENTION, usually in the form of police warnings and restraining orders."

If you get a restraining order, expect it to be violated. Ellen Sorokin reports that "According to a 1997 Justice Department Study, three out of every four protection orders issued across the country each year will be routinely violated at some point by a jilted lover, an angry ex-husband, or an obsessed admirer. But only a small fraction of those violators will ever be punished.

In Virginia, for example. more than 7,200 protective orders have been authorized...since July 1977. Yet in Northern Virginia alone...only 15 persons were charged with violating protective orders, and only five were convicted, according to Virginia Supreme Court records."

Stalkers are more likely to obey a restraining order if they understand that they have a lot to lose by violating it, for example, a man who has a good job and standing in his community may not be willing to risk the embarrassment of being arrested for violating the order. On the other hand, a man who is obsessed or delusional or impervious to social pressures may be more willing to ignore the RO. Stalkers who have had a long, emotional relationship with their victims tend to ignore ROs more often than stalkers who are strangers. Stalkers who are mentally ill also violate judicial orders frequently.

All other things being equal, a restraining order that is obtained early in the crime is more likely to be effective than one that is obtained after months or years of criminal activity, when both the stalker's habits and his thought patterns are more entrenched.

View with suspicion any stories you hear about what happened before stalking was a crime, or when ROs were not aggressively enforced. Try to find out what has happened recently in the location where you live, to determine how the police, courts, and prosecutors are currently handling stalking cases and RO violations.

If the stalker violates a RO in some jurisdictions, you can get a lifetime RO against him.

In some places where basic stalking is simply a misdemeanor, violating an RO is a felony.

In some places, violating a RO subjects the stalker to harsher penalties for stalking than would be possible without the RO.

If you file for a restraining order, you should be very specific about what is included in it. Schaum and Parrish suggest that you might want to include any or all of the following:

- Placing you under surveillance or following you
- Approaching or confronting you in a public place or on private property.
- Appearing at your workplace or residence.
- Entering onto or remaining on property owned, leased, or occupied by you, even when you are not on the premises.
- Contacting you by telephone, pager, or fax
- Sending mail or electronic communications to you.
- Placing an object on, or delivering an object to property owned, leased, or occupied by you.

If you have obtained a restraining order, make multiple copies so you can keep one at home, one at work, one in your car, and carry one with you at all times. Take a copy to your local police department, and other nearby police departments, including the one that would respond to any emergency at your work. Find out if there is a way to register your restraining order so that all the police or judges in the county or the state will know about it; if not, send your own copies as widely as you can.

It may cost you money to file for a restraining order. If you do not have it, you might be able to save money by not using a lawyer or by asking for help from a battered women's organization. Even if you are not a victim of domestic violence, the people who run battered women's shelters have a lot of expertise about obtaining restraining orders with very little money, and will be happy to share this information with you. They may also be able to help you find low or no cost legal advice.

When your stalker violates the restraining order, you will have to prove that the violation occurred.

Find out in advance whether the police will actually take the stalker to jail when he violates the restraining order. Sometimes the police promise to arrest him, but "arrest" may mean just giving him a citation!

Reid Meloy, one of the country's foremost experts on stalking, said, at a recent Threat Assessment Conference, that in looking at the results of 14 studies in restraining orders, 8 of them showed success, 4 mixed results, and 2 negative results. But these studies generally mix domestic violence and stalking; at least one study focused solely on stalking, and found ROs were negative.

To estimate the chances of violence after a RO is served, Meloy suggests asking:

What is the history of violence against the victim?

How preoccupied or obsessed is he?

How has he reacted to ROs before?

What is the intensity of his feelings for her?

How effective will enforcement of the RO be?

There is a probable link between dominance expressed in the prior sexual relationship (sadism, handcuffs, control, etc.) and his later violence as a stalker.

In conclusion, whether to obtain a restraining order or not is an intensely personal, and intensely important, decision. Weigh the pros and cons of your particular case carefully with a number of different people before making your decision.

❖ *"Should I move? Change jobs?"*

This is not an easy question to answer. For some, it is the best way to be safe; for others, it is expensive, time consuming, emotionally exhausting, and not guaranteed to work.

If you decide to stay where you are, you might want to take immediate steps to make your home address less available to someone who is searching for it.

If you decide to move, be very sure to take all the precautions you possibly can, and make arrangements in advance so that your new address will not appear anywhere unless you have determined it is safe.

If you are thinking about moving, "disappearing," or becoming very, very hard to find, you should read *How to Lose Anyone Anywhere*, by Michael Scott. It has a wealth of information about how to be sure, really, really sure, that you won't be found or followed.

If you are thinking about changing jobs, consider how hard or easy it would be for the stalker to find you again. If you are a professional who will be easily traceable, perhaps through state licensing or professional organizations, changing jobs is unlikely to help much, but if you can change the type of work you are doing as well as the location, you have a better chance of losing him in the process.

If you are being stalked at work by someone associated with your work, changing jobs might help. Perhaps your company can change your work location, and help to keep the new location a secret from the stalker.

If you decide to leave your job because of stalking, see if your employer or union will give you an arrangement in which you leave your job, get a financial settlement from your old employer, and outplacement assistance.

If you are self employed, you might be able to change a lot about your work, such as its mailing address, to keep it very separate from your home.

❖ *"How does the stalker find me?"*

Stalkers use 4 methods, primarily, to find information about their victims:

1. Talking. Just talking with friends, family, co-workers, and others. One stalker pretended to be a realtor interested in selling his target's house; he went to neighbors, and found out lots of personal information about his target's family.
2. Public records
3. Semi-public resources such as using Internet resources, or paying a private investigator to find information
4. Surveillance

A stalker can find your current address by searching major credit bureaus, if he has your social security number and any address you have lived at for about the last 7 years. While it is illegal to obtain credit information without the consent of the individual—not that stalkers would be stopped by that restriction—it is actually not illegal to obtain the "header information" and other non-credit information from the credit bureau. Address information is in the header. Credit bureaus update new address information as soon as you fill in the new address section of your credit card bill when you pay it.

There are on-line searches that, given just a name, comb every public record available in the US, and provide address histories for everyone with that name.

Cellphone records show both the number called and the number doing the calling. These records are relatively easy to get.

If the stalker has a rough idea of where you own property, he can go to the county assessor's office to get your residential address.

Most states allow any citizen full access to court files pertaining to civil, criminal, and domestic cases. These may involve residential addresses, business addresses, dates of birth, or social security numbers.

In most states, drivers' licenses and vehicle registration information are public; if not public, they are often easily available.

A huge amount of information is available on the Internet. An archive called Deja-News will find any messages you have ever posted to any newsgroup. A plethora of search engines, from a military personnel locator to various people-locators, promise to find information on people. Generally, these are entirely legitimate and are used for benign purposes. However, they can become dangerous sources of personal information for stalkers.

Many companies use prison inmates for computer data entry work. A woman filed a lawsuit as a result of harassment from an incarcerated rapist in a Texas prison who got her name and other personal information from a product questionnaire she had filled out in exchange for coupons and free samples. Many states use prison labor for computer entry of various public records, including motor vehicle registrations. Federal prisoners perform data entry for the Internal Revenue Service. "Some of our best computer operatives were sex offenders" John Benestante, director of state prison industries for Texas, said, quoted in Snow's book.

Finally, some stalkers read books like this one. We at AWARE would like to keep it out of the hands of stalkers. Please do your part, and keep your copy where it won't be stolen if your stalker gets into your home.

❖ *"I have kids. Is there anything special I should do?"*

Being responsible for the safety of your children as well as yourself is sometimes an additional burden, but it is also a tremendous incentive.

You need to teach them basic safety habits and drills as soon as you think they are old enough, such as how to call 911 and not to open the door to anyone without checking with you first.

Unfortunately, it probably isn't possible to completely avoid having any contact at all with your ex if you have to hand the kids back and forth, but you can do a lot to minimize the amount of contact, and to maximize your safety during those contacts.

Some women partially solve this problem by sticking to a pre-defined schedule for exactly when and where the kids are exchanged, so that phone calls each time to make arrangements aren't necessary. Some enlist the assistance of family or friends in the exchanges, so that they never need come into direct contact with their abuser. Other women arrange to exchange the children only in very public places, where they feel safer.

If you have to drop off and pick up the kids yourself, here are some general rules that will help keep you and your children alive:

1. Plan ahead.
2. Do not get any closer to him than absolutely necessary (and keep something between you whenever possible).
3. Have an escape route (or two).
4. Keep a close eye on him (especially his hands).
5. If he produces a weapon, get out of there FAST!

Let's look at how these rules could be applied. Suppose you have a child you are going to drive to drop off, and your ex has been threatening you (but not your child). Arrange for the exchange to take place in a very public place, such as the parking lot of a supermarket, a busy fast food restaurant, or a busy, open gas station. (A parking lot when nobody is around would be a poor location, as would be either your home or his.) Another part of planning ahead is to arrive with your doors locked and windows up.

Before you suggest a particular place for the dropoff or pickup, drive to it at the time of day you would be using it. Scope out escape routes, places to hide, and think about what he might do to take advantage of the physical location, and what you might do. Know the neighborhood well enough to know several places you could drive in an emergency. On the day of the child exchange, try to let him get there first, so he will already have parked, and you can orient your car accordingly. Remember the section on car and parking safety? Those principles apply here, too.

When you drive up, never park head in. Either back into a parking space moderately far away, or, if he is parked head in, you can drive up and stop behind him so that your car blocks his. The point is to arrange the relative positions of the cars so that if you have to drive away quickly, you can do so easily, and he will have some difficulty in following, or at least he will have to make a turn to do so, which will slow him down.

To keep away from him, you can just let an older child out of your car to go to his, and then drive away.

If your child is young enough to need you to get out with her, leave your car's engine running. Ask him to get out of his car to meet you; you don't want to get close to him while he is in his car where a weapon could easily be concealed. As soon as he gets out of his car, start watching his hands. Hands with anything in them that could be used as a weapon may signal danger. Hands in pockets where you can't see them may signal danger.

Try to keep something between you, such as the body of your car, until you can see that his hands are empty. If you can't keep in that position, at least be aware of other cars or objects you could use for cover if necessary.

If you see him produce or brandish a weapon, don't hesitate for an instant—RUN, preferably to your car to get out of there, but behind other cars or anything that will shield you! Even if you have a gun, you probably should not produce it until you and your child are behind cover. If he has threatened your child, or you have reason to believe that he intends to harm your child as well as you, then be sure your child stays with you. But if you are certain that you are his only intended victim, it might be better for your child, as well as you, for you to move away from her, leaving her behind cover if possible. I know that seems unthinkable, but do you really want your daughter at your side or in your arms when that depraved man starts shooting at you? Remember that by acting quickly to save yourself, you will be ensuring that your child will grow up with the presence of a loving mother, instead of only the vague memory of a murdered one.

That's the worst case scenario. Now let's go back to considering the normal scenario, where you don't see any weapon.

If you don't see a weapon, turn over your child and any toys, bags, etc. quickly. Now HIS hands will be full, and unlikely to go for a weapon.

Don't use these meetings to discuss anything that can possibly be handled another way. You don't want to risk getting drawn into a discussion that may quickly escalate to anger. Get back to your car as soon as you can, and drive away.

Obviously, this kind of scenario has thousands of variations, with and without cars, with multiple children, and in many different places. However, if you follow the 5 general rules, you should make it through every drop-off and pick-up alive, and, if you are subtle about it, your ex will never even know that you are utilizing a whole set of defensive strategies!

❖ *"I may be a target for a celebrity stalker. What can I do?"*

Remember that you don't have to be a celebrity to have a celebrity stalker. Anyone in the public eye, from local politicians to rock stars can attract this kind of unwanted attention. So can people in any profession, but particularly the helping professions: medicine, nursing, social work, therapy, and so on.

The good news for you is that if you can put preventive measures in place before the stalker gets underway, they are very likely to be effective in protecting you.

Robert Bardo, the stalker who eventually murdered actress Rebecca Schaeffer, first tried to pursue Tiffany and Debbie Gibson, but found that he could not get close to either of them. He even followed Debbie Gibson to New York, but could not find out where she lived. Gavin de Becker says, "When a target proves inaccessible, everybody assumes that a fanatic fan will simply opt for another time and another place. It's not so. If a public figure avoids an encounter once or twice, that's often the end of it for them. Their pursuer will likely focus on another target."

So, the earlier in the stalking that you can identify the fact that you have a problem and react appropriately to it, the more likely your "fan" will simply give up.

Your stalker is likely to have some major mental problems, and probably isn't getting adequate, or any, treatment for them. It is extremely difficult, in today's climate, to force treatment on anyone, so there isn't much you can do, except be alert for any signs of threats of suicide—then you might be able to get him committed.

Linden Gross says, "Ironically, a mentally ill person who threatens to take his own life will get quicker response from mental health services than if he threatens to take someone else's. If you pose a danger to yourself, treatment is almost guaranteed."

The good news is that, in general, mentally ill people don't commit as many crimes as normal people do. The bad news is that the minority who do commit crimes have a great tendency to be repeat offenders, and to be extremely dangerous.

If your stalker is getting psychiatric treatment, of course you are not entitled to any details about it, but if you can find out the names of the doctors or therapists who are treating him, you can at least remind them that they have a duty to warn you if your stalker poses a hazard of great bodily harm to you. (This is called the Tarasoff warning, after a famous case in which a student named Tiana Tarasoff was murdered by her stalker, another student, and was given no warning by the university psychologist who was trying to treat the stalker.)

❖ *"What can the police and others do to help me?"*

Police "intervention" in stalking situations is a subject of much debate in the law enforcement community. Everyone agrees that police should investigate stalking cases, and arrest stalkers who violate ROs. What isn't so clear is whether police should, for example, "talk" to a known stalker to try to discourage him from continuing his activities. Sometimes this works, sometimes it seems to be a factor in escalating the stalker's activities.

The LAPD Threat Management Unit uses "vertical management" of stalking cases, in which one detective has the case forever, even after the stalker gets out of prison and starts the harassing behavior again. The detective will contact the victim very frequently while the case is active, and occasionally when it is inactive; if the suspect is known, he will contact the suspect, too. Interviews with the suspect are always conducted face to face, never by phone, but may be at the stalker's home, place of work, police station, or other location.

The LAPD TMU says that ROs are "extremely effective" if they are followed up properly. In California, violating a restraining order in a stalking situation is a felony. Violations MUST be handled right away, with arrest and detention.

The Domestic Violence Response Team in Colorado Springs, CO has developed a program that helps them identify and manage cases of very high risk domestic violence offenders. It is a team approach that includes victim advocates, a detective, and a case worker if kids are involved. They got a "blanket order" that allowed sharing of otherwise unsharable information across agencies. They give victims alarm systems, 911 cellphones, telephone recorders, and so on. They get very high bonds, $30,000 for stalking, as compared to $800 for a misdemeanor. This seems like an excellent program that more police departments should know about. Perhaps you can persuade your police department to call them for advice.

Nashville, TN serves virtually all stalking restraining orders within 48 hours! Nashville will also prosecute cases with or without the victim's cooperation. One stalker made 27 phone calls to his victim in violation of a restraining order, and the judge sentenced him to 10 days for each call!

So, there is a lot that other people can do to help keep you safe, and to get your stalker off the street!

❖ "I'm on a tight budget. How can I afford safety?"

No matter how much money you have, absolute safety can't be bought. The former Beatle George Harrison and his wife Olivia were attacked by a stalker, in their home, despite the presence of a private security force. It was the prompt, decisive actions of the couple themselves, including Olivia swinging a lamp at the intruder and knocking him out, that saved them from very likely being killed.

Fortunately for us ordinary folk, living in a state of relaxed awareness doesn't cost a dime, and is the one single thing that is most likely to save your life.

Although many of the suggestions thus far in this book involve buying some kind of equipment or paying for some kind of lessons, you don't have to spend a lot of money to be safe. You can pick and choose your investments in safety very carefully.

One way to gradually increase your security without spending a bundle is to make safety-conscious decisions when you are making normal purchases. Moving to a new place and having new locks installed? This would be a good time to decide on the better quality of lock instead of the cheapest, and to get 3-inch screws instead of 2-inch to install them. The incremental cost is small, but the increase in safety is great.

Some security methods actually save you money, such as getting rid of easily identifiable vanity license plates on your car.

Here are some other suggestions for staying safe without emptying your bank account.

- ## Gifts

Ask your friends and family for safety-oriented gifts for holidays and birthdays. Drop hints for a cellphone or paper shredder. For expensive items, a few friends or relatives might want to go in together to buy them.

- ## Use professionals who are just learning

If you cannot afford professional assistance (for anything from legal advice to a massage to relieve stress), find out if there is a school for those professionals near you. They might have programs where you can get services from students in training, supervised by their teachers.

- ## Free books

Don't want to spend a fortune on books? Visit a public library and ask for help finding the books you want, or similar ones.

- ## Low cost computer access

For free or low-cost computer access, visit a public library.

You can rent a computer to use at home instead of buying one, but this is cost-effective only if you are going to use it for a very short time.

Ask computer-savvy friends if you can use their computer (or their help doing so) when you need to search the web for information.

Some services are much cheaper during evenings or on weekends.

- ## Cheap phones, or substitute phones

Cellphones for emergency use only are available for low (or no) monthly fees. Some companies have prepaid phones, where you buy a cellphone and a card, good for a year. You get some minutes free each month, with no monthly fee.

Sometimes local agencies or women's organizations will lend cellphones to women in danger.

CB radios are cheaper than cellphones. You don't always know who is answering your call, but at least you can broadcast a message for help, particularly if you are in a car.

As a last resort, get a non-working cellphone (perhaps from your phone company's repair shop). Keep it in your car, so you can appear to be using it to call for help. Seeing you "on the phone" might deter someone, at least temporarily.

• Cheap window safety

Don't want to pay for fancy window locks? If you have windows that slide up and down, drill a hole about 6 inches above the lower window, and insert a big nail or wooden dowel to prevent the window from being raised more than that distance.

• Free safety audit

Most police departments offer a free home security review, in which they point out possible deficiencies in locks, lighting, and so on. (Be sure to tell them that you need security against more than the common burglar.)

• Use videos

If you want to take a particular course but cannot afford it and cannot get it on a sliding fee scale, try some videos on the same subject. While not as effective as a personal lesson, they are much cheaper and are often more effective than books for many techniques.

• Use student services

If you are a student, your school probably has many resources for you to tap, from registrars who may let you change your student ID number, to security guards who will walk with you, to free Internet access.

See if there is a women's organization on campus with services regarding safety. Offer to be a case they can use to create services for stalking victims, if none exist already.

• Share with friends

Find folks in similar circumstances to yours at a stalking victims' support group or domestic violence support group, and suggest sharing the cost of some resources that you all can share.

Get a group of your friends together for a "work party" to install security devices in your home, or to do other safety-related chores.

• Women's shelter or crisis hot line

You may think of these resources only for rape survivors or people in abusive relationships, but the people who run these sorts of facilities are often knowledgeable about things a bit outside their main area of expertise, and their services are generally free or very low cost. If you don't fit their guidelines, be sure to ask them for referrals to other people and organizations.

• Cheap legal advice

To find a low or no cost lawyer, contact some local battered women's shelters or other women's organizations, even if you are not a battered spouse. You might also call Legal Aid, or contact a local law school to see if they have law school clinics that offer free assistance. Some states have state-funded offices such as state women's commissions, domestic violence coordinators, district attorneys, and victim witness advocates to provide help, information, and referrals.

• **Use nonprofit agencies**

In every community there are non-profit groups that provide information and assistance at no or low cost.

AWARE is one such organization, and, although we do not have the resources to teach classes in every part of the country, we can provide services to individuals by telephone toll free 877-67-AWARE (877-672-9273), email (info@aware.org), and our web site (www.aware.org).

• **Awareness is free!**

It doesn't cost anything to open your eyes and ears and look around you to see, really see, your environment. It doesn't cost a penny to stay alert, particularly at times when you know your stalker may be around. Thinking about what he might do, and what you would do in response, is the best kind of mental rehearsal for getting through a tough situation. And it is absolutely free!

Interlude 5: What would you do?

You put up with a lot during your marriage. You never told anyone about the beatings, or the marital rape. Your husband kept a stranglehold on the family finances—you couldn't even write a check. He was equally controlling of your time, and he was so mean to your friends that they gradually started staying away from you. But it was worth it, because of your son, the light of your life.

Things were sort of ok for quite a few years, but when your son got to be about 6 years old, your husband started beating him, too. You tried to make him stop by threatening to divorce him, but he would just say, "You do that, and I'll kill you both." You weren't sure if he meant it, but you couldn't take the chance.

After a particularly awful beating, you suddenly realized that your husband might very well kill your son if you didn't leave. Feeling sick and scared, you finally took your son and got out, managing to get to as far as the home of a former girlfriend, who took you both in for a few months.

Almost immediately, your husband managed to track you down. He phoned a hundred times a day. When nobody would answer the phone, he would come over and pound on the door and scream that he was going to kill you, but he was always gone before the police could arrive. You are pretty sure he started a fire in a trashcan near your temporary home.

What would you do?

This is a very tense, dangerous situation for you, your son, and your friend. Some help from people experienced in domestic violence situations is definitely called for, as is a crash course in protecting yourself.

If the police and social service agencies are not being helpful, you must insist that they do better. Remind them, "Lots of people in my situation have been killed. I don't intend to be one of them! My son is not going to be one of them!" Tell them exactly what you want them to do to help you.

Meantime, know that you must keep yourself safe so that you can keep your son safe. Some things in this book that you would never have thought you would do suddenly seem very reasonable, considering the very real danger to you both.

13 Mistakes To Avoid

Remember the stalking victim who said that it took her a long time for her to learn that it is impossible to reason with a stalker? Every stalking victim could tell you stories of what they did wrong, as well as what they did right. Learning from the mistakes of others is an important way to avoid going down the same long, dangerous way yourself.

If you aren't a stalker's target, but are trying to help someone who is, it is equally valuable to know what NOT to do.

❖ Mistakes stalking victims make

• Ignoring warning signs

It is a bad mistake to ignore the early warning signs that say "this guy seems a little strange." Not all stalkers seem peculiar at first, but if you pick up any uncomfortable feelings, pay attention to them.

Putting up with extreme jealousy or possessiveness or physical violence in a relationship is also a mistake.

• Feeling pity

Going on a "pity date" with someone who pesters you, but who you aren't interested in getting to know better, is a recipe for future trouble.

Feeling pity for the stalker may be difficult, particularly if he is a former boyfriend or husband. Don't let these feelings prevent you from taking defensive measures, or calling the police when they are needed.

• Using ineffective strategies

Thinking you can reason with him is the number one mistake most stalking targets make.

Spending a long time trying to persuade him to stop is particularly ineffective. If he doesn't hear your "no" early on, it is time to move on to other strategies.

Not informing other people, thinking "I can take care of this situation by myself," is a common problem, sometimes magnified by being afraid of looking foolish if you confide your situation to friends or police.

Negotiating with the stalker is always a poor idea. Anything more than a single, explicit statement that you do not want a relationship with him will be taken as a negotiation, that is, as an invitation for the stalker to continue his behavior. As long as you talk, no matter what you say, he will continue both talking and stalking.

• Minimizing the danger

It is tempting to believe that if he hasn't made an explicit threat, you aren't really in danger, but it isn't true.

Saying, to yourself or others, "It can't get any worse than this," is just wishful thinking, and may keep you from preparing to deal with the situation if it does worsen.

Saying, to yourself or others, "I'm not going to change the way I live just because someone is stalking me," also prevents you from making the changes that are necessary to ensure your safety.

• **Rewarding the stalker**

DeBecker warns against inadvertently sanctioning the stalker's behavior by saying something soft and non-committal, such as "I'm just not ready for a relationship right now." He will view this as "I will be ready for a relationship with you eventually, so keep trying." Don't say, "I don't want a boyfriend right now." He will interpret this as meaning that you will want a boyfriend some time in the future, and it might be him.

Don't inadvertently rewarding the stalker's behavior by having some contact with him, such as finally picking up the phone after he has called you 50 times and gotten your answering machine, or answering the door after the 100th time he rang your doorbell. You just taught him that it takes at least 50 calls or 100 rings to get in touch with you, and next time he'll gladly try even harder, maybe 100 phone calls or 200 doorbell-rings.

Don't inadvertently rewarding the stalker by having indirect contact with him, such as having a friend call him or visit him in an effort to make him stop. He will view these emissaries as messengers from you, and he will think this is good, regardless of what your friend says. Visits from police, private detectives, or other professionals MAY have the desired effect, but this is not guaranteed.

• **Underestimating him**

It is easy to underestimate the tenacity of stalkers. An obsessed stalker will violate any trust, disregard any rule, and break any law.

• Reducing vigilance

It is extremely tempting to let down your guard because you have taken a lot of precautions, or because your stalker is, at the moment, in jail. You need to live your life as if he might get out at any time.

• Revenge or retaliation; getting even

Do not try to turn the tables by stalking your stalker. It is always a mistake to let your anger turn into aggression in ways that are unsafe for you, or illegal.

Don't try to beat the stalker at his own game; by trying to follow him, frighten him, hurt him, or create a booby-trap for him. All of these things can incur tremendous liability for you, resulting in monetary damages or even criminal proceedings against you!

Never play "get even" games with the stalker, trying to follow him to find out who he is, or trying to intimidate him into ceasing his harassment. The stalker may view these activities as an indirect contact with you, which is what he wants.

❖ *Mistakes police and the legal system make*

• Underestimating the severity of this crime

Not taking stalking seriously.

Releasing stalkers on low bonds, particularly if they have repeated violations.

Waiting for the stalking to reach "serious" levels, such as an explicit threat. This simply gives more time for the stalker's obsession to deepen.

Short prison sentences, particularly if the stalker has repeat violations.

• Rewarding stalkers with the victim's presence

Forcing victims, particularly celebrities, into a face to face confrontation in court with their stalkers. This cements the stalker's relationship with the victim, as in the case of Madonna's stalker, who derives status in prison from his "relationship" with her.

• Minimizing the value of self-defense training

Not encouraging victims to learn self-protection, including firearms if necessary, from appropriately qualified sources.

Believing that a rape-oriented self-defense course is all a stalking victim needs, because it will make her "feel better."

• Too many police or prosecutors

Having a different detective or prosecutor work with a single stalking case at each point in the process (arraignment, pretrial motions, trial) makes it very difficult for the victims to learn what is going on, and to provide helpful information in a timely way.

• Too few referrals

Thinking their organization can do it all. It is natural for people helping stalking victims to think that their service is the most important, but no one group can do everything. Police, prosecutors, non-profit agencies, and other groups should constantly inform women of other sources of information and assistance.

• Mishandling restraining orders

Not enforcing restraining orders quickly and with consequences that are real to the stalker.

• Not keeping victims informed

Not informing when stalkers are released. The local police department should be informed, as well as the victim. More corrections departments should use VINE, which stands for Victim Information and Notification Everyday. VINE is a system that automatically monitors the jail's computer to keep track of inmates. When an inmate is released, or there is a change in custody or court date, the computer automatically calls anyone registered with the VINE program (such as the victim) and notifies them. The calls continue for 24 hours, unless the person calls back with the shutoff code. People who register with VINE give only a name and phone number, not an address. VINE makes most calls within 10 minutes, and is no additional burden on the already overworked correctional staff. If the correctional facility you are dealing with does not use VINE, find out why, and whether they would use it if they could buy it. Then get creative about finding the funds to put this kind of system in place.

❖ *Mistakes friends and family make*

• Not taking it seriously

Saying "Oh, isn't that cute!" "He's just in love with you!" "You should be flattered by all that attention," or "I wish he'd call me instead of you."
Not protecting your personal information adequately.

• **Trying to deal with the stalker themselves**

Challenging the stalker.
Threatening the stalker.
Trying to reason with, convince, or frighten the stalker into stopping.
Communicating with the stalker in any way.

14 Dealing with the Stress

The stress of being stalked can be very intense, particularly if you are feeling isolated and afraid. Most stalking targets report that they feel a negative change in their health and mental attitude as a direct result of their ordeal.

Linden Gross, the founder of the non-profit organization Stalking Survivors' Sanctuary & Solutions, says, "Victims respond not with a single reaction, but with a progression of emotions akin to Elizabeth Kubler-Ross's five stages of loss: denial, bargaining, guilt, anger, and then acceptance. Because they participate, however unwillingly, in the crime, they also experience depression, anxiety, and fear."

Here are some things that may help you cope:

- Keep yourself fit. Eat well, even if you have to force yourself, and exercise.
- Treat yourself well. Don't deny yourself the little things that give you pleasure. A bubble bath or seeing a new movie can provide a much-needed lift.
- Don't isolate yourself from family and friends. You may think you are protecting them, but you need their concern and support.
- Use the medical and mental health resources available to you. That's what they are there for!

When people are afraid, particularly for a long period of time, they will do almost anything to make the fear stop. Stalkers know this, and use that knowledge to manipulate you. Protect yourself by learning how to be alert without being fearful—a good self-defense class can start to show you how. It will truly empower you (not just make you feel good), and will provide you with some new ways to protect yourself.

Feeling depressed? Notice that your memory isn't as good as it used to be? Are you anxious, irritable and easily startled? Is your sleep disturbed, even when your stalker leaves you alone for the night? Do you have trouble concentrating, or making decisions? Are you feeling hopeless and helpless? Are you emotionally "numb"? Do you have trouble making decisions? Do you feel like your thinking or your body has slowed down? Do you suffer from unexplained pain, indigestion, fatigue, dry mouth, or dizziness? Do you find yourself getting angry easily, crying a lot, or going on buying sprees? These are all signs of stress.

Many stalking victims find relief by talking with mental health professionals who are familiar with stress disorders. Remember, depression is a disease, and it is treatable just like many other diseases.

Find yourself thinking about suicide? You aren't alone. In recent study, nearly a quarter of the stalking victims interviewed said they had thought about it. Get some professional help, and you will get through this difficult time.

Take good care of yourself in ways other than those related to safety. Eat well, get exercise, and spend enjoyable time with friends and family. You are under tremendous stress, and these things are very important in coping with it.

Poetry and the arts give many people a way to express what is going on in their lives.

Melita Schaum puts it accurately and concisely: "As much as possible, let neither the stalker nor fear of him rule your life. Take action, and fill your days with the people, places, and things that give you comfort and joy."

Afterword

Congratulations—you've just done a difficult and terribly important thing. You've started taking responsibility for your safety!

When you think, "I don't want to do all those self-protection things, because I don't want my stalker to have that much control over my life," remember that he has more control over you now, by making you afraid and keeping you that way. Your choice is either:

1.   Keep doing exactly what you have been doing (for example, go to and from work at the same time every day). You will feel afraid because, quite realistically, you are in danger—he knows when and where to find you, or he can easily find out.

or

2.   Take some modest steps to increase your safety (such as varying your comings and goings). You may be annoyed at doing so, but you will be less afraid, because you are in less danger, since you are in control, making it harder for him to find you.

Which are you going to do?

Like being raped, having a critical illness, being hurt in a serious accident, or losing a beloved family member, stalking is a major, life-changing event that happens to you against your will. Being stalked changes your life suddenly, dramatically, and forever, but it isn't all bad. You become stronger, and learn things about your own capabilities that you never knew.

Read the section on "Relaxed Awareness" again. If you start training yourself to spend most of your waking hours in that state, you will be aware, alert to problems before they occur, and ready to respond to them, but not constantly fearful and stressed out.

Nothing helps like talking with other people who have been where you are. Find a support group, or contact people in the organizations listed in the appendices of this book.

Though there may be storms ahead, knowledge and preparation will prevail over mindless violence. As Louisa May Alcott, the author of *Little Women*, said, "I am not afraid of storms, for I am learning to sail my ship." Learn to sail yours, and you will not be afraid of the storms ahead.

Be well. Stay safe.

Appendix A: Organizations and Web Sites

Web sites come and go very quickly, so please understand if some of these links have changed or disappeared by the time you try them. Please let AWARE know of other web sites that you find helpful, so we can include them in future editions of this book.

If you don't have a computer with an Internet account, any public librarian should be able to help you access these resources. If you would prefer to write or call for information, that information has been included wherever possible.

Stalking, and More

http://www.aware.org
AWARE, Arming Women Against Rape and Endangerment, is a national non-profit group that provides information and training for women to enable them to avoid, resist, or repel crimes ranging from minor to major. Not everything is on the web; special information available on stalking.
AWARE
PO Box 242
Bedford MA 01730-0242
781-893-0500
Toll free: 877-67-AWARE

http://www.try-nova.org/
The National Organization for Victim Assistance (NOVA)
Web site has some interesting info, such as "Running the Talk Show Gauntlet"
1730 Park Road NW
Washington · DC
202-232-6682
Fax: 202-462-2255

http://www.ncvc.org/
The National Center for Victims of Crime site has a huge amount of information for victims of all kinds of crimes, and for people who don't want to be one. From statistics to strategies, even has talk show guidelines for crime victims.
National Victim Center
2111 Wilson Blvd., Suite 300
Arlington VA 22201
800-394-2255

http://www.aclu.org/privacy/
The ACLU has an interesting web site dealing with privacy issues; it includes some good info on safeguarding SSNs, medical information, and other kinds of information.
American Civil Liberties Union
125 Broad Street, 18th Floor
New York, New York 10004-2400
212-549-2585

http://www.ojp.usdoj.gov/vawgo.
US Office of Justice Programs, Violence Against Women program. This site contains their annual reports to Congress, with a large amount of information and statistical detail about stalking and domestic violence.
Violence Against Women Office
810 7th Street, NW
Washington, DC 20531
202-616-8894

http:// www.wirelessfoundation.org
A foundation that supplies free emergency cellphones for women at high risk of violence.

Specifically Stalking

http://www.demographics.com/Publications/AD/98_ad/9803_ad/ad980311.htm
Some statistics on stalking.

http://www.weq.gov.bc.ca/stv/stalking/default.html#toc
Lots of good information from the Canadian government for stalking victims.

http://www.uic.edu/depts/safetynet/stalking.html
Do's and Don't list, plus links to other sites.

http://www.soshelp.org/
Survivors of Stalking, an organization that provides support for stalking victims; good advice from those who have been there.
Survivors Of Stalking
PO Box 20762
Tampa FL 33622

http://www.apbonline.com/safestreets/1998/11/07/stalktips_01.html
More info for stalking victims in a news article.

http://www.smalltime.com/notvictims/stalking.html
Links to other stalking resources.

http://www.fiu.edu/~victimad/st.htm
Links to other stalking resources.

www.stalkingbehavior.com/
Detailed descriptions and analysis of stalking behavior, with a good reference list.

http://www.stalkingvictims.com/
Stalking Victim's Sanctuary; offers many suggestions such as ways to regain a feeling of control in your life; has a national online support group for victims.
Stalking Survivors' Sanctuary & Solutions
P.O. Box 400
Angels Camp, CA 95222
877-782-5533

http://www.zdnet.com/anchordesk/story/story_1781.html
General news story on stalking.

http://www.antistalking.com
The AntiStalking Website, has some good advice and detailed information on stalkers; includes some descriptions of famous and not-so-famous stalking cases.

http://francieweb.com/stalked/
A stalking victim's own page, with info about staying safe and stories from various stalking victims.

http://www.madcapps.com/Writings/faqabout.htm
NetGuide Mazagine stalking law and guidelines. Though a little dated, there is some good material here.

Legal, Police, Privacy, and Related Issues

http://www.nvc.org/law/statestk.htm
State stalking laws, from the National Center for Victims of Crime.

http://www.epic.org/privacy/consumer/legal.html
Information about state privacy laws.

www.privacyrights.org
Privacy Rights Clearinghouse; mostly for California residents, but some info is for everyone.
1717 Kettner Ave. Suite 105
San Diego, CA 92101
619-298-3396
619-298-5681
Email: prc@privacyrights.org

http://www.ci.dover.nh.us/police/Domestic%20Violence/informat.htm
This is from a New Hampshire police department; it includes stalking info, and a videotape for stalking victims.

http://www.nashville.net/~police/risk/index.htm
Nashville police web site with quizzes you can take to rate your likelihood of being raped, murdered, or robbed.

http://www.ilj.org/stalking/
Institute for Law and Justice web site; has links to other online sites with stalking info, and info for cyberstalking.
Institute for Law and Justice
1018 Duke Street
Alexandria, VA 22314
703-684-5300

Cyberstalking, Safety on the Internet

http://www.cyberangels.org/
Excellent general information on using the Internet safely.
CyberAngels
PO Box 480901
Kansas City, MO 64148

http://whoa.femail.com/
Women Halting Online Abuse. A useful site with info about protecting yourself online.

http://www.cybercrime.gov/cyberstalking.htm
A government report on cyberstalking.

http://www.ncvc.org/special/cyber_stk.htm
Cyberstalking page of the National Victims Center.

http://www.crimelibrary.com/criminology/cyberstalking/
Overview article on cyberstalking.

http://www.cyberguards.com
CyberGuards site has a section on cyberstalking.

Self-Protection Tools and Skills

http://www.ayoob.com/cat1.html
Police Bookshelf, source for Persuaders and other defensive tools.
Police Bookshelf
PO Box 122
Concord NH 03302-0122
800-624-9049

http://www.awsda.org
American Women's Self-Defense Association.
713 N. Wellwood Avenue
Lindnhurst NY 11757
631-225-6262
Toll free: 1-888-StopRape

http://www.defendyourself.net
Another source for Persuaders

http.//www.bamm.org, or http://www.bedrock.com:80/dc-impact/chapters.htm
Impact / Model Mugging

http://www.rad-systems.com/
Rape Aggression Defense (RAD) system of physical training
498-A Wythe Creek Rd.
Poquoson, VA 23662
757-868-4400

http://www.nwmaf.org/
National Women's Martial Arts Federation.

http://www.nrahq.org/safety/education/basictraining.html.
NRA's firearms courses.
NRA
11250 Waples Mill Road
Fairfax VA 22030
202-828-6000
Toll free: 800-392-8683

http://www.martialartsresource.com/firearms.htm
http://www.shooters.com
Pages that leads to a number of firearms schools.

http://www.gunhoo.com
To find firearms schools, search for TRAINING. This site also has a section for women.

http://www.womenandguns.com
Women&Guns magazine.
267 Linwood Avenue
PO Box 488 Station C
Buffalo NY 14209-9930
716-885-6408

http://www.ssdd.com/
Scotti School of Defensive Driving

http://www.racesearch.com/resources/drvschls.html
This site has links to a number of driving schools, defensive as well as racing.

http://www.autoguide.net/schools/driving.shtml
A directory of national driving schools

http://www.nsc.org/training/index.cfm
National Safety Council index to defensive driving schools.

Credit Bureaus and Information Services

http://www.equifax.com/
CBI-Equifax
PO Box 105496
Atlanta, GA 30348
800-997-249

http://www.experian.com/
Experian (formerly TRW)
P.O. Box 2104
Allen, TX 75013-2104
Toll free: 888-397-3742

http://www.lexis-nexis.com/lncc/about/removal_copy(1).html
The form you can fill out to have personal information removed from
their records.
Lexis-Nexis
P.O. Box 933
Dayton, Ohio 45401-0933
937-865-6800
800-227-9597

http://www.tuc.com/
Trans Union
Consumer Disclosure Center
P.O. Box 1000
Chester, PA 19022
800-888-4213.

Appendix B: Sample Stalking Log

Date:_____ Time:_____

Location: _____

Stalking activity:_____

_____

_____

_____

Witnesses:_____

_____

Victim's actions in response: _____

_____

_____

_____

Bibliography

Alcott, Louisa May, A *Long Fatal Love Chase*, Dell Publishing, 1995, ISBN 0-440-22301-6.

In 1866, two years before she published *Little Women*, Alcott wrote this novel of passionate obsession that was "too sensational" to be published during her lifetime.

Ayoob, Massad. *In the Gravest Extreme*. Police Bookshelf, 1980, ISBN 0-936279-00-1.

The must-read classic for anyone considering a firearm for self-defense.

Browning, Wilt. *Deadly Goals*. St. Martin's Paperbacks, 1997, ISBN 0-312-96220-7.

A true-crime account of college football star Pernell Jefferson, the women he abused, and the one he finally stalked, raped, and murdered.

deBecker, Gavin. *The Gift of Fear*. Little, Brown, 1997, ISBN 0-316-23502-4.

Not just about stalking, this book is becoming a classic in the field of general self-protection for women.

Douglas, John and Olshaker, Mark. *Obsession, The FBI's Legendary Profiler Probes the Psyches of Killers, Rapists, and Stalkers and Their Victims and Tells How to Fight Back*. Pocket Books, 1998, ISBN 0-671-01704-7.

A fascinating historical account, mostly about serial killers.

Evans, John. *The Child Stalker.* 1995, Covenant House Books, ISBN 0-925591-36-X.

A former FBI agent describes the hunt for the man who abducted and killed two Nebraska boys.

Fine, Robert. *Being Stalked: A Memoir.* Chatto & Windus, Random House UK, 1997, ISBN 0-7011-6685-1.

A British professor gives his account of being stalked by a female student.

Gross, Linden. *Surviving a Stalker.* Marlowe & Co, 2000, ISBN: 1-56924-604-1.

Excellent description of the problems of stalking, and how to deal with many of them.

Hardy, Bo. *Defensive Living, When Defensive Driving, Diets and Exercise Aren't Enough to Keep You Alive and Well.* Defensive Living Press, 1992, ISBN 0-9633237-9-2.

Though written for people trying to avoid mugging and rape, this no-nonsense book has many excellent tips for making your life style a defensive one.

Kamir, Orit, *Every Breath You Take, Stalking Narratives and the Law,* University of Michigan Press, 2001, ISBN 0-472-11089-6.

Traces how ideas of stalking have evolved from ancient mythology to contemporary film and social science.

Lardner, George. *The Stalking of Kristin.* Penguin Books, 1997, ISBN 0-451-40731-8.

Powerful, Pulitzer-prize winning account of his daughter's murder, and how "the system" failed to help her.

Markman, Ronald and LaBrecque, Rob. *Obsessed—The Stalking of Theresa Saldana*. New York: William Morrow and Company, 1994, ISBN 0-688-10970-5.

This is one of the celebrity stalking cases that resulted in the first anti-stalking law.

May Hayes, Gila, *Effective Defense*, Firearms Academy of Seattle, 1994, ISBN 1-885036-01-9.

Superb information about attitude, pepper spray, Persuader/Kuboton, and much more.

Meloy, J. Reid, editor. *The Psychology of Stalking, Clinical and Forensic Perspectives*. Academic Press, 1998, ISBN 0-12-490560-9.

A collection of academic articles for those who want to read about research on stalking.

Mullen, Paul E., Pathe, Michele and Purcell, Rosemary. *Stalkers and Their Victims*. Cambridge University Press, 2000, ISBN 0-521-66950-2.

An excellent overview of stalking, from the perspective of psychiatrists and psychologists who treat stalkers; this book summarizes the findings and limitations of current research, and includes many case studies.

Orion, M.D., Doreen. *I Know You Really Love Me, A Psychiatrist's Account of Stalking and Obsessive Love*. Dell Publishing, 1997, ISBN 0-440-22599-X.

Stalked for years by an erotomanic female patient, this is the well-written story of a psychiatrist's personal and professional journey to understand stalking.

Peck, Richard, *Are You in the House Alone?*, Puffin Books, 1976, ISBN 0-14-130693-9.

A novel for teens about a girl who is being stalked.

Rich, Curt. *Drive to Survive!* MBI Publishing, 1998, ISBN 0-7603-0525-0. Defensive driving tactics and tips.

Schaum, Melita and Parrish, Karen. *Stalked; Breaking the Silence on the Crime of Stalking in America.* Pocket Books, 1995, ISBN 0-671-88710-6. Information-packed book, from stories to what-to-do, to resources.

Scott, Michael. *How to Lose Anyone Anywhere: The Stalking Victims Rodamap to Safety.* Stealth Publishing, 1996, revised 1999, Library of Congress Number TX-4-180-204.
Excellent information if you really want to start over without leaving a trace; good general information on phones, mail, and other aspects of protecting your privacy.

Snow, Capt. Robert L. *Stopping A Stalker, A Cop's Guide to Making The System Work for You.* Plenum Press, 1998, ISBN 0-306-45785-7.
Mostly stories about stalkers and their victims.

Snortland, Ellen. *Beauty Bites Beast: Awakening the Warrior Within Women and Girls.* Trilogy Books, 1998, ISBN 1-891290-00-2.
About Impact self-defense training and the personal empowerment to be gained by knowing how to fight back!

Sorokin, Ellen. "Anti-Stalking Laws Usually are Unable to Protect Targets." *Washington Times*, April 17. 2000.
Useful article about the effectiveness of stalking laws.

Spence-Diehl, Emily. *Stalking: A Handbook for Victims.* Learning Publications, 1999, ISBN 1-55691-161-0.
Slim volume of good information, including sample stalking logs.

Stange, Mary Zeiss and Oyster, Carol K. *Gun Women, Firearms and Feminism in Contemporary America.* New York University Press, 2000, ISBN 0-8147-9760-1.
Not about self defense, but a interesting exploration of the relationship between firearms and women, from many perspectives; it asks "Can a woman be a feminist and a gun owner too?"

Wright, Cynthia. *Everything You Need to Know About Dealing With Stalking.* Rosen Publishing Group Inc., 2000, ISBN 0-8239-2841-5.
Excellent book, specifically for teenagers.

Printed in the United States
88892LV00004B/100/A